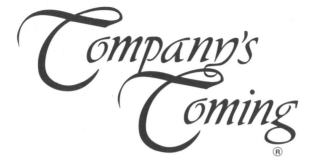

Diabetic Cooking

Jean Paré

www.companyscoming.com
visit our website

We gratefully acknowledge the following suppliers for their generous support of our Test and Photography Kitchens:

Broil King Barbecues	Hamilton Beach® Canada	Proctor Silex® Canada
Corelle®	Lagostina®	Tupperware®

Diabetic Cooking

First Printing April 2007

Library and Archives Canada Cataloguing in Publication
Paré, Jean, date
Diabetic cooking / Jean Paré.
(Original series)
Includes index.
ISBN 978-1-897069-28-8
1. Diabetes—Diet therapy—Recipes. I. Title. II. Series: Paré, Jean, date- Original series.
RC662.P36 2007   641.5'6314   C2006-905634-X

Published by
Company's Coming Publishing Limited
2311 – 96 Street
Edmonton, Alberta, Canada T6N 1G3
Tel: 780-450-6223 Fax: 780-450-1857
www.companyscoming.com

Table of Contents

Appetizers &
Beverages

Breads &
Muffins

Breakfasts

Desserts

Lunches

Main Dishes

Salads

Side Dishes

Soups

The Company's Coming Story

Jean Paré (pronounced "jeen PAIR-ee") grew up understanding that the combination of family, friends and home cooking is the best recipe for a good life. From her mother, she learned to appreciate good cooking, while her father praised even her earliest attempts in the kitchen. When Jean left home, she took with her a love of cooking, many family recipes and an intriguing desire to read cookbooks as if they were novels!

"never share a recipe you wouldn't use yourself"

In 1963, when her four children had all reached school age, Jean volunteered to cater the 50th Anniversary of the Vermilion School of Agriculture, now Lakeland College, in Alberta, Canada. Working out of her home, Jean prepared a dinner for more than 1,000 people, which launched a flourishing catering operation that continued for over 18 years. During that time, she had countless opportunities to test new ideas with immediate feedback—resulting in empty plates and contented customers! Whether preparing cocktail sandwiches for a house party or serving a hot meal for 1,500 people, Jean Paré earned a reputation for good food, courteous service and reasonable prices.

As requests for her recipes mounted, Jean was often asked the question, "Why don't you write a cookbook?" Jean responded by teaming up with her son, Grant Lovig, in the fall of 1980 to form Company's Coming Publishing Limited. The publication of *150 Delicious Squares* on April 14, 1981 marked the debut of what would soon become one of the world's most popular cookbook series.

The company has grown since those early days when Jean worked from a spare bedroom in her home. Today, she continues to write recipes while working closely with the staff of the Recipe Factory, as the Company's Coming test kitchen is affectionately known. There she fills the role of mentor, assisting with the development of recipes people most want to use for everyday cooking and easy entertaining. Every Company's Coming recipe is *kitchen-tested* before it's approved for publication.

Jean's daughter, Gail Lovig, is responsible for marketing and distribution, leading a team that includes sales personnel located in major cities across Canada. In addition, Company's Coming cookbooks are published and distributed under licence in the United States, Australia and other world markets. Bestsellers many times over in English, Company's Coming cookbooks have also been published in French and Spanish.

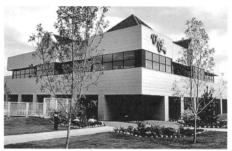

Familiar and trusted in home kitchens around the world, Company's Coming cookbooks are offered in a variety of formats. Highly regarded as kitchen workbooks, the softcover Original Series, with its lay-flat plastic comb binding, is still a favourite among readers.

Jean Paré's approach to cooking has always called for *quick and easy recipes* using *everyday ingredients.* That view has served her well. The recipient of many awards, including the Queen Elizabeth Golden Jubilee medal, Jean was appointed a Member of the Order of Canada, her country's highest lifetime achievement honour.

Jean continues to gain new supporters by adhering to what she calls The Golden Rule of Cooking: *"Never share a recipe you wouldn't use yourself."* It's an approach that works—*millions of times over!*

Foreword

When a family member has diabetes, all too often it has meant cooking one meal for him or her, and cooking a different meal for the rest of the family. No longer. Now the entire family can enjoy tasty recipes and benefit from a well-balanced eating plan with *Diabetic Cooking*. What could be better? Treat your family to great-tasting, kitchen-tested recipes that have the added perks of being low in fat and sugar.

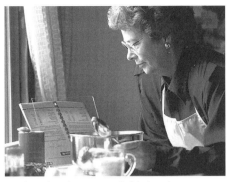

Over the years many of my readers have asked for a diabetic cookbook, so I had thought of creating one well before my husband Larry was diagnosed with Type 2 diabetes. With today's focus on healthy eating, I admit to baking less, if only to provide fewer temptations around the house.

Many people with diabetes miss their desserts, but they can fit treats into their daily meals in consultation with a dietitian. Check out the Desserts section for Strawberry Banana Frozen Yogurt, French Pastry Dessert or Lemon Angel Tower.

From the first page to the last, *Diabetic Cooking* is designed to bring you great-tasting food. Try Crispy Barbecue Chips with Black Bean And Corn Salsa as a snack or appetizer for a party, or whip up some Honey Wheat Bread for lunch with Couscous Seafood Salad. Fix Jambalaya or quick and easy Creamy Garlic Penne for supper. How about Turkey Cutlets with Mushroom Sauce with a side dish of Cheese Spirals or Stuffed Tomatoes? When you feel like celebrating a special occasion, concoct a batch of out-of-this-world Brownies or Cherry Chocolate Dessert. Share them and be prepared for rave reviews from all!

During development of this book, we convened a focus group of people of all ages with diabetes to sample our recipes. They held us up to their high standards, making sure this book would meet with your approval too. After all, food that's good for you still needs to taste good enough to eat! We also wish to thank the dedicated volunteers and staff of the Juvenile Diabetes Foundation for their valued input and encouragement.

Whether you have diabetes, are cooking for someone who has diabetes, or are just interested in a healthier lifestyle, you'll be glad you picked up your copy of *Diabetic Cooking*!

Jean Paré

Each Recipe has been analyzed using the Canadian Nutrient File from Health and Welfare Canada, which is based upon the United States Department of Agriculture (USDA) Nutrient Data Base.

Margaret Ng, B.Sc. (Hon.), M.A.
Registered Dietitian

Diabetic choices have been assigned based upon the nutrition information per serving stated.

Vera C. Mazurak, Ph.D.
Nutritionist

About diabetes

When someone has diabetes, their blood has too much glucose—a type of sugar—because their body isn't processing it properly. The body receives glucose from digestion of carbohydrates such as those found in grains, fruits and vegetables, and milk. The liver also produces glucose that travels into the blood stream.

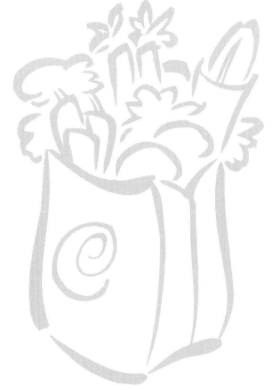

Under healthy conditions, the pancreas produces enough insulin to enable glucose to enter cells and be used as fuel. People with Type 1 (or insulin-dependent) diabetes have a severe lack of insulin because their pancreases produce little or none at all. In order to maintain normal blood glucose levels, they need to take insulin injections and control their intake of fats and carbohydrates. People with Type 2 (or non insulin-dependent) diabetes still produce insulin, but not enough, or their bodies do not use it efficiently. They may be able to manage their disease with diet alone or with a combination of diet, pills and/or insulin injections.

Without treatment, symptoms of diabetes may include increased thirst and urination, fatigue, vision changes and weight loss. In the long term, diabetes can damage the eyes, kidneys, nerves, heart and circulation system. Being physically active and maintaining a healthy body weight are keys to good living for everyone, but critical for those with diabetes.

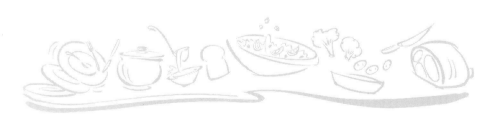

About diabetic eating

Diabetic Cooking *is a cookbook filled with enticing, easy-to-prepare food. It follows the theory that dietary guidelines for people with diabetes are the same for everyone: eat a wide variety of nutritious food in moderation.* **Every person with diabetes needs to consult with a dietitian to determine his or her personal eating plan.**

Performance-enhancing foods

No foods are forbidden—limiting the consumption of alcohol, salt, fat and sugar doesn't necessarily mean *eliminating* those items. Just like putting the wrong kind of gasoline in your car affects performance, fueling your body with poor food choices does the same thing. The cost of eating "premium fuel" doesn't have to be a premium price. Some cuts of meat may seem pricey, but not when you consider that a portion of steak is only 4 oz. (113 g), rather than the overly-large 8 oz. (225 g) portion you're likely to get at a restaurant. Likewise, fresh fruits and vegetables fluctuate in price, so buy them in season and then compare the cost to their processed cousins-in-a-can. Convenience foods are often high in fat, salt and sugar, so stay clear of them—that way only your wallet will grow fatter!

Sweet dreams

Advice about sugar consumption for people with diabetes has changed over the years. Small quantities of sugar that don't cause a quick peak in blood sugar levels are now allowed. A large soft drink or chocolate bar will have a lot of concentrated sugar, but a small piece of chocolate or candy will have a lesser effect on blood glucose levels.

Smart snacking

Fresh fruit and ice cream are simple desserts or snacks that, in small quantities, have lower fat than regular cheese and crackers. Foods like nuts, salami and olives are also high in fat, so low-fat cheese, dips and breads would be preferable as fill-ins between meals. If you can, find yummy add-ons like a wonderful low-fat salad dressing from our Salads section to go with "free foods" (those without quantity restrictions), such as green and leafy vegetables.

Lightly starched

While starchy foods may cause blood sugar spikes, they are still carbohydrates, which are something every body needs. Complex carbohydrates with fibre (generally foods which have not been highly processed) are more nutritious and better at keeping blood glucose levels on an even keel.

Decoding dietary info

Nutrition Information

For each recipe in *Diabetic Cooking*, we have
provided nutrition information, which tallies
calories, fat (including cholesterol and saturated
fats), carbohydrates, fibre, protein and sodium.
These values include all the ingredients listed in
the recipe except those stated as "optional" or
"for garnish." If a range of measurements is
given, the smaller amount is analyzed. Variations
of recipes listed underneath the analysis and
ingredient substitutions given in brackets
have not been analyzed.

Diabetic Choices (Beyond the Basics)

Each recipe in this revised edition of *Diabetic Cooking* contains
the diabetic choice values for the updated Beyond the Basics meal
planning guide. Beyond the Basics groups together foods that are
similar in carbohydrate content. The names of the categories have
been changed to better reflect the foods contained in the group.
For example, Starches has become Grains and Starches, whereas
Sugars has become Other Choices to better reflect the sweets and
snack foods in the group. Although the allowed size or amount of
different food within a particular group may vary, each food in that
group will have the same approximate composition of carbohydrates,
protein, fat and calories. If no choices are listed, it means that
the serving size suggested for that food does not have enough
carbohydrates to constitute a choice in any category.

For people on insulin who require precise carbohydrate counting,
the nutritional information giving total grams of carbohydrate and
dietary fibre will provide useful guidelines.

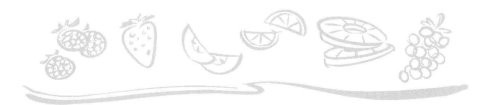

Ingredients at work

Artificial Sweeteners: When testing the recipes in *Diabetic Cooking*, we did not use artificial sweeteners, with the exception of a few recipes where a large amount of sugar would have been required or because we wanted to provide some recipes where they could be substituted for sugar or honey.

Fats: We chose to use canola or olive oil instead of margarine where we could. In some recipes, margarine or butter was better for taste, but we limited the amount. Butter can be used moderately, but it is an animal fat and contains cholesterol. Where possible, we used non-stick cookware or no-stick cooking spray to reduce the fats and oils used.

Meats: All the meat we used was trimmed of fat prior to cooking. We also chose lean cuts such as boneless, skinless chicken breasts or beef sirloin.

Milk: Our test kitchen staff used skim milk unless specified, since it has an equal amount of calcium and approximately the same amount of nutrients as 1%, 2% or whole milk, without any of the animal fat.

Egg Substitute: Most of our recipes call for only one or two eggs. For recipes using more than two eggs or those considered to be primarily egg dishes, we've used a lower cholesterol egg substitute. For certain recipes we chose to use an egg substitute because the recipe already had other saturated fats. If preferred, avoid using egg yolks to reduce fat and cholesterol (the whites contain high-quality protein without the fat).

Cheese: We used light sharp Cheddar cheese, part-skim mozzarella or light Parmesan cheese product to lower the fat content without compromising the taste.

Yogurt: These recipes were tested using plain and flavoured non-fat yogurt. With minimal effort, you can make Yogurt Cheese, page 75, and use as a substitute for cream cheese.

Cooking Methods: We recommend baking, grilling, steaming, poaching and stir-frying to reduce the amount of fat needed to cook an item.

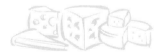

If you have any questions about how these recipes, or any other food, can fit into the diet of someone with diabetes, please talk to your doctor or dietitian.

Take-Along Booster

When your blood sugar is plummeting and you need a quick fix fast,
keep this sweet, tropical-tasting treat at the ready (see Tip, below).

Container of vanilla frosting	16 oz.	450 g
Almond flavouring	1/4 tsp.	1 mL
White corn syrup	1/3 cup	75 mL
Finely chopped dried apricots	1 1/2 cups	375 mL
Icing (confectioner's) sugar	3 cups	750 mL
Flake coconut	1 cup	250 mL

Icing (confectioner's) sugar (optional)
Flake coconut (optional)

Combine frosting and flavouring in large bowl.

Measure corn syrup into small bowl. Microwave on high (100%) for 30 seconds or warm in small saucepan on low. Stir in apricots until well coated. Add to frosting mixture. Stir well.

Stir in icing sugar and coconut. Knead with hands to combine well. Turn out onto flat surface. Knead, adding icing sugar if required to prevent sticking, until smooth. Measure into 1/2 tbsp. (7 mL) portions. Roll into balls.

Roll in additional icing sugar or coconut. Wrap individual balls in plastic wrap. Freeze. Makes about 52 balls.

1 ball: 83 Calories; 1.1 g Total Fat (0.7 g Sat., 1.7 mg Cholesterol); 10 mg Sodium; trace Protein; 19 g Carbohydrate; trace Dietary Fibre

CHOICES: 1 Other Choices

tip   Boosters are high-sugar snacks designed to jump-start your sugar levels when they plummet, so don't substitute the sugar-free version of flavoured gelatin. However, using the lower-fat products is a good idea. These boosters are meant to be frozen in individual portions and taken along with you **for emergencies only**. They are not meant to be included as part of your daily meal plan.

Boosters

Sweet Cereal Booster

This s'more-like treat won't let you down when the going gets tough (see Tip, page 10).

Light smooth peanut butter	1/2 cup	125 mL
Corn syrup	1/4 cup	60 mL
Miniature marshmallows	3 cups	750 mL
Vanilla	1/2 tsp.	2 mL
Corn flakes cereal	5 cups	1.25 L

Melt peanut butter and corn syrup in large saucepan on low. Stir in marshmallows until just melted. Do not overcook. Remove from heat.

Stir in vanilla and cereal until well coated. Press firmly into greased 9 x 9 inch (22 x 22 cm) pan. Cool to room temperature. Cut into 24 bars. Wrap individual bars in plastic wrap. Freeze. Makes 24 bars.

1 bar: 84 Calories; 2.3 g Total Fat (0.4 g Sat., 0.1 mg Cholesterol); 96 mg Sodium; 2 g Protein; 15 g Carbohydrate; trace Dietary Fibre

CHOICES: 1/2 Grains & Starches; 1/2 Other Choices; 1/2 Fats

Loopy O Booster

This fruity little bar will carry you through when you're feeling slow on the go (see Tip, page 10).

Margarine	2 tbsp.	30 mL
White corn syrup	1/3 cup	75 mL
Package of fruit-flavoured gelatin (jelly powder), your favourite (not sugar-free)	3 oz.	85 g
"O"-shaped fruity cereal (such as Fruit Loops)	4 cups	1 L

Melt margarine in large saucepan on medium. Stir in corn syrup and jelly powder. Heat and stir until boiling and jelly powder is dissolved. Remove from heat.

Quickly stir in cereal to coat. Mixture will be very sticky, so work fast. Press firmly into greased foil-lined 8 x 8 inch (20 x 20 cm) square pan. Chill just until set. Cut into 18 bars. Wrap individual bars in plastic wrap. Freeze. Makes 18 bars.

1 bar: 74 Calories; 1.4 g Total Fat (0.3 g Sat., 0 mg Cholesterol); 60 mg Sodium; 1 g Protein; 15 g Carbohydrate; trace Dietary Fibre

CHOICES: 1 Other Choices

Crispy Barbecue Chips

These don't have to be in wedges; they can be cut into irregular shapes. Pile in a bowl for a snack with friends. Try with Black Bean And Corn Salsa, page 15.

Spicy barbecue sauce	1/3 cup	75 mL
Olive oil	2 tsp.	10 mL
Sesame seeds	2 tsp.	10 mL
Garlic powder	1/8 tsp.	0.5 mL
Whole wheat flour tortillas (10 inch, 25 cm, size)	4	4

Combine first 4 ingredients in small dish.

Brush both sides of tortillas with barbecue sauce mixture. Cut each into 10 wedges. Arrange wedges in single layer on large greased baking sheet. Bake on bottom rack in 350°F (175°C) oven for 8 minutes. Turn wedges. Bake for 8 minutes until crispy and browned. Makes 40 chips.

2 chips: 42 Calories; 0.8 g Total Fat (0.1 g Sat., 0 mg Cholesterol); 77 mg Sodium; 1 g Protein; 7 g Carbohydrate; trace Dietary Fibre

CHOICES: 1/2 Grains & Starches

Pictured on page 17.

Herb Dip

Good with any cut-up vegetables. The flavour is much better when made a day ahead.

Non-fat plain yogurt	1 cup	250 mL
Non-fat salad dressing (or non-fat mayonnaise)	1/4 cup	60 mL
Parsley flakes	2 tsp.	10 mL
Chopped fresh chives (or 2 tsp., 10 mL, dried)	1 tbsp.	15 mL
Dried whole oregano, crushed	1/2 tsp.	2 mL
Dried sweet basil	1/2 tsp.	2 mL
Dried tarragon leaves, crushed	1/8 – 1/4 tsp.	0.5 – 1 mL
Dry mustard	1 tsp.	5 mL
Salt	1/2 tsp.	2 mL
Granulated sugar	1/2 tsp.	2 mL

Combine all 10 ingredients in small bowl. Cover. Chill for at least two hours to blend flavours. Makes 1 1/8 cups (280 mL).

1 tbsp. (15 mL): 12 Calories; 0.1 g Total Fat (trace Sat., 0.3 mg Cholesterol); 110 mg Sodium; 1 g Protein; 2 g Carbohydrate; trace Dietary Fibre

CHOICES: None

Spicy Mexi-Bean Dip

Make this recipe to accompany Fresh Tomato Salsa, page 16.
Serve both with Crispy Barbecue Chips, page 12.

Cooked (or 1 can, 19 oz., 540 mL) black beans, drained and rinsed	1 1/2 cups	375 mL
Diced jalapeño pepper, ribs and seeds removed (see Tip, page 105)	1 tbsp.	15 mL
Salsa	1/4 cup	60 mL
Light sour cream	1/4 cup	60 mL
Grated light Monterey Jack cheese	1 1/2 cups	375 mL

Mash beans with fork or masher in medium bowl until broken up. Add next 3 ingredients and 1/2 of cheese. Spoon into shallow 1 quart (1 L) casserole. Sprinkle remaining 1/2 of cheese on top. Bake, uncovered, in 350°F (175°C) oven for 20 minutes or until bubbly. Makes 2 cups (500 mL).

2 tbsp. (30 mL): 67 Calories; 3.6 g Total Fat (2.4 g Sat., 10.3 mg Cholesterol); 118 mg Sodium; 4 g Protein; 5 g Carbohydrate; 1 g Dietary Fibre

CHOICES: None

Pictured on page 17.

Simple Tuna Spread

Serve with a variety of lower-fat crackers. Or take for lunch along with crackers, bread or fresh vegetables. For more flavour, add a little more teriyaki sauce.

Finely chopped red onion	2 tbsp.	30 mL
Can of white tuna, packed in water, drained and broken into chunks	6 oz.	170 g
Teriyaki sauce	4 – 6 tsp.	20 – 30 mL

Combine all 3 ingredients in small bowl. Chill for 1 to 2 hours to blend flavours. Makes 1 cup (250 mL).

1 tbsp. (15 mL): 17 Calories; 0.4 g Total Fat (0.1 g Sat., 5.0 mg Cholesterol); 70 mg Sodium; 3 g Protein; trace Carbohydrate; trace Dietary Fibre

CHOICES: 1/2 Meat & Alternatives

Variation: Omit teriyaki sauce and add 2 tbsp. (30 mL) non-fat herb and garlic-flavoured cream cheese and 2 tsp. (10 mL) low-sodium soy sauce.

Crab Appetizers

These little morsels are good hot or cold. Serve with seafood cocktail sauce.

Finely chopped imitation crabmeat	2 cups	500 mL
Fine dry bread crumbs	3/4 cup	175 mL
Creamed horseradish	1 tsp.	5 mL
Chopped green onion	1/2 cup	125 mL
Finely chopped red or yellow pepper	1/2 cup	125 mL
Chopped fresh parsley (or 1 tsp., 5 mL, flakes)	1 tbsp.	15 mL
Dry mustard	1 tsp.	5 mL
Salt	1/2 tsp.	2 mL
Freshly ground pepper, sprinkle		
Dried sweet basil, crushed	1/4 tsp.	1 mL
Dried whole oregano, crushed	1/8 tsp.	0.5 mL
Garlic powder (optional)	1/8 tsp.	0.5 mL
Frozen egg product, thawed (see Note)	1/2 cup	125 mL

Combine first 12 ingredients in large bowl. Stir well.

Stir in egg product. Cover with plastic wrap. Chill for 1 hour for bread crumbs to moisten. Roll rounded tablespoonfuls (15 mL) mixture into thirty-four 1 1/2 inch (3.8 cm) balls. Arrange on greased baking sheet. Bake in 350°F (175°C) oven for 10 minutes until firm and golden brown. Makes 34 balls.

2 balls: 51 Calories; 0.7 g Total Fat (0.1 g Sat., 8.4 mg Cholesterol); 296 mg Sodium; 5 g Protein; 7 g Carbohydrate; trace Dietary Fibre

CHOICES: 1/2 Grains & Starches; 1/2 Meat & Alternatives

Pictured on page 18.

Note: 4 tbsp. (50 mL) = 1 large egg

Paré Pointer

Knock knock.
Who's there?
Beth.
Beth who?
Beth let me in or I'll blow your houth down!

Black Bean And Corn Salsa

Put in the whole jalapeño for more of a hit. Use with Crispy Barbecue Chips, page 12.

Can of black beans, drained and rinsed	19 oz.	540 mL
Chopped red onion	1/2 cup	125 mL
Chopped fresh cilantro	1 tbsp.	15 mL
Diced jalapeño pepper, ribs and seeds removed (see Tip, page 105)	1 tbsp.	15 mL
Lime juice	1 tbsp.	15 mL
Ground cumin	1/4 tsp.	1 mL
Chili powder	1/4 tsp.	1 mL
Large tomato, seeded and chopped	1	1
Garlic clove, minced	1	1
Can of kernel corn, drained	12 oz.	341 mL
Salt	1/2 tsp.	2 mL

Combine all 11 ingredients in medium bowl. Cover. Chill for at least 2 hours to blend flavours. Makes 4 cups (1 L).

1/4 cup (60 mL): 39 Calories; 0.2 g Total Fat (trace Sat., 0 mg Cholesterol); 167 mg Sodium; 2 g Protein; 8 g Carbohydrate; 1 g Dietary Fibre

CHOICES: None

Pictured on page 17.

 tip Although there is no meat in vegetarian dishes, beans and chick peas provide a lot of protien. Kidney beans contain more protein than meat and are very rich in vitamins.

Fresh Tomato Salsa

Brightly coloured and very fresh in flavour. A finely chopped jalapeño or other hot pepper could be added if you like it hot! Will keep for 1 day covered in refrigerator, but it will have much more liquid.

Seeded, diced Roma (plum) tomatoes	2 cups	500 mL
Finely diced red onion	1/4 cup	60 mL
Finely diced green pepper	1/4 cup	60 mL
Garlic cloves, minced	2	2
Salt	1/4 tsp.	1 mL
Freshly ground pepper, generous sprinkle		
Chopped fresh sweet basil (or 2 tsp., 10 mL, dried)	3 tbsp.	50 mL
Chopped fresh chives	1 tbsp.	15 mL
Red wine vinegar	1 tbsp.	15 mL
Chopped fresh cilantro (optional)	3 tbsp.	50 mL

Combine all 10 ingredients in medium bowl. Let stand at room temperature for at least 1 hour to blend flavours. Makes 2 1/2 cups (625 mL).

1 tbsp. (15 mL): 3 Calories; trace Total Fat (0 g Sat., 0 mg Cholesterol); 17 mg Sodium; trace Protein; 1 g Carbohydrate; trace Dietary Fibre

CHOICES: None

Pictured at right.

Variation: Substitute balsamic vinegar for red wine vinegar for a deeper taste.

1. Crispy Barbecue Chips, page 12
2. Piña Colada Smoothie, page 25
3. Black Bean And Corn Salsa, page 15
4. Spicy Mexi-Bean Dip, page 13
5. Fresh Tomato Salsa, above

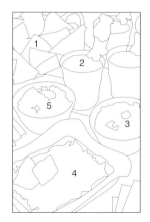

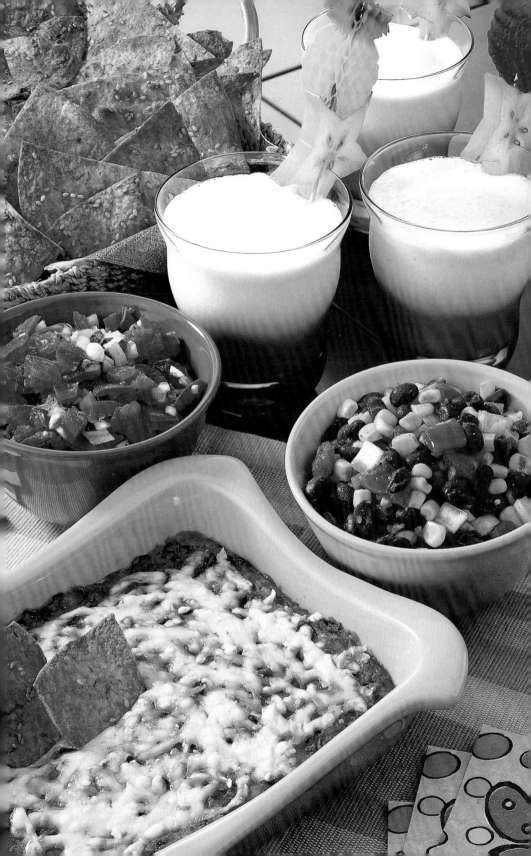

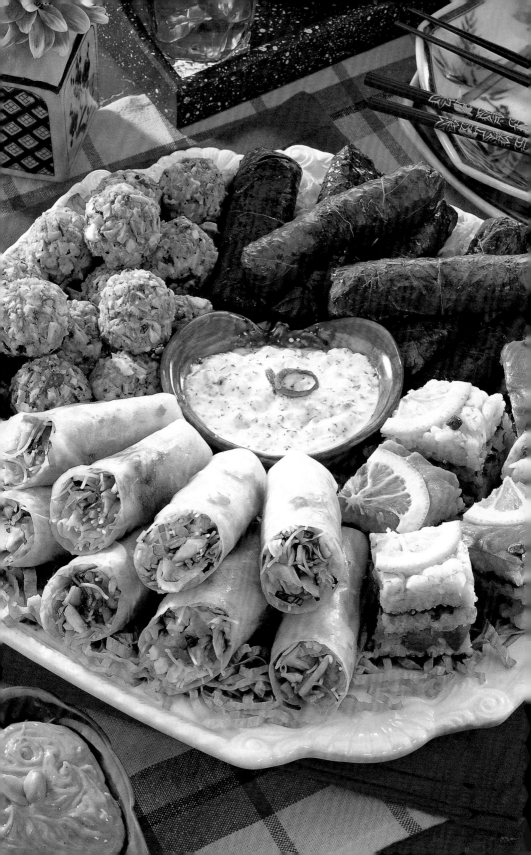

Smoked Salmon Mousse

Spread on stoned wheat crackers or baguette slices.

Tomato juice	1/2 cup	125 mL
Envelope of unflavoured gelatin	1/4 oz.	7 g
Can of red salmon, drained, skin and round bones removed	7 1/2 oz.	213 g
Green onions, cut into 1 inch (2.5 cm) pieces	2	2
Non-fat creamed cottage cheese	3/4 cup	175 mL
Non-fat plain yogurt	1/2 cup	125 mL
Liquid smoke	1/8 tsp.	0.5 mL
Lemon juice	2 tsp.	10 mL
Freshly ground pepper, sprinkle		

Combine tomato juice and gelatin in small saucepan. Let stand for 5 minutes. Heat and stir on low until gelatin is dissolved. Set aside.

Process remaining 7 ingredients in food processor, scraping down sides as necessary, until smooth. Add gelatin mixture through chute. Mix well. Pour into lightly greased plastic-lined 2 1/2 cup (625 mL) mold or deep bowl. Cover with plastic wrap. Chill for several hours until firm. To serve, turn out and remove wrap. Makes 2 1/2 cups (625 mL).

1 tbsp. (15 mL): 13 Calories; 0.3 g Total Fat (0.1 g Sat., 1.9 mg Cholesterol); 45 mg Sodium; 2 g Protein; 1 g Carbohydrate; trace Dietary Fibre

CHOICES: None

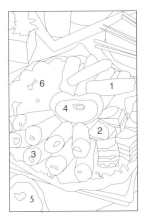

1. Stuffed Grapevine Leaves, page 23
2. Sushi Layers, page 22
3. Salad Rolls, page 20
4. Fresh Yogurt Sauce, page 21
5. Peanut Sauce, page 20
6. Crab Appetizers, page 14

Salad Rolls

*These are so good. Keep for up to 2 hours in refrigerator
under a damp paper towel and wrapped in plastic.*

Water	1/3 cup	75 mL
Thick teriyaki sauce	2 tbsp.	30 mL
Low-sodium soy sauce	1 tbsp.	15 mL
Cornstarch	2 tsp.	10 mL
Fish sauce (optional), see Note	1/4 – 1/2 tsp.	1 – 2 mL
Shredded lettuce, lightly packed	2 cups	500 mL
Chopped fresh bean sprouts	1 cup	250 mL
Green onion, thinly sliced	1	1
Fresh sweet basil leaves, cut chiffonade (see Tip, page 135)	12	12
Fresh pea pods, chopped (optional)	1/3 cup	75 mL
Grated carrot	1/3 cup	75 mL
Chopped imitation crabmeat	3/4 cup	175 mL
Rice vermicelli	1 oz.	28 g
Hot water		
Rice paper wrappers (8 inch, 20 cm, size)	12	12
Warm water		
PEANUT SAUCE		
Light smooth peanut butter	1/2 cup	125 mL
Non-fat plain yogurt	1/2 cup	125 mL
Medium-hot curry paste (see Note)	1 1/2 tsp.	7 mL
Chili paste (optional)	1/4 tsp.	1 mL
Lime juice	1 1/2 tsp.	7 mL
Finely chopped peanuts, for garnish		

Combine first 5 ingredients in small saucepan. Heat and stir on medium until boiling and thickened. Cool thoroughly.

Combine next 7 ingredients in medium bowl. Set aside.

Break vermicelli into small pieces in small bowl. Cover with hot water. Let stand for 3 minutes until softened. Drain. Rinse with cold water. Drain thoroughly. Add to lettuce mixture. Toss.

(continued on next page)

Soak each rice wrapper in warm water in 9 inch (22 cm) pie plate for 2 minutes until soft. Place packed 1/3 cup (75 mL) lettuce mixture across one side of center, leaving 1 inch (2.5 cm) piece of wrapper on each side uncovered. Drizzle 2 tsp. (10 mL) sauce over filling. Fold sides of wrapper over filling. Roll tightly over filling. Press gently at seam to seal. Place on serving platter. Cover with damp paper towel to keep from drying out. Repeat with remaining wrappers and filling. Cut each roll in half crosswise to serve. Makes 12 rolls or 24 half rolls.

Peanut Sauce: Whisk all 6 ingredients together in small bowl until smooth. Let stand at room temperature for 10 minutes to blend flavours. Makes 1 cup (250 mL) sauce. Garnish with peanuts.

1 full roll with 2 tsp. (10 mL) sauce: 82 Calories; 2.5 g Total Fat (0.4 g Sat., 3.5 mg Cholesterol); 237 mg Sodium; 3 g Protein; 11 g Carbohydrate; trace Dietary Fibre

CHOICES: 1/2 Grains & Starches; 1/2 Fats

Pictured on page 18.

Note: Both fish sauce and curry paste are available in Asian section of grocery store.

Fresh Yogurt Sauce

Substitute Yogurt Cheese, page 75, for the yogurt and texture will be thicker—great for a dip or to serve on baked potatoes.

Grated English cucumber, with peel	1/2 cup	125 mL
Salt	1/4 tsp.	1 mL
Low-fat plain yogurt	1 cup	250 mL
Garlic clove, minced	1	1
Chopped fresh mint leaves (or parsley)	2 tbsp.	30 mL

Combine cucumber and salt in small bowl. Let stand for 10 minutes. Pour into sieve. Squeeze cucumber until most of liquid is gone. Return to bowl.

Add remaining 3 ingredients. Stir gently. Cover. Chill for 1 hour to blend flavours. Makes 1 1/2 cups (375 mL).

1 tbsp. (15 mL): 7 Calories; 0.2 g Total Fat (0.1 g Sat., 0.7 mg Cholesterol); 35 mg Sodium; 1 g Protein; 1 g Carbohydrate; trace Dietary Fibre

CHOICES: None

Pictured on page 18.

Sushi Layers

No bamboo mat or special technique required for these!
They cut well and are easy to hold in your hands.

Water	4 1/2 cups	1.1 L
Rice vinegar	1/3 cup	75 mL
Granulated sugar	1/4 cup	60 mL
Salt	1 tsp.	5 mL
Short grain (or pearl) rice	2 1/4 cups	550 mL
Rice wine (sake) or dry sherry	1/4 cup	60 mL
Medium lemons, sliced paper-thin and seeded	2	2
Small capers, drained and rinsed	1 tbsp.	15 mL
Package of paper-thin slices smoked salmon	3 oz.	85 g
Small cooked shrimp	8 oz.	225 g
Nori sheets	4	4
Thinly sliced cucumber, with peel (about 1/2 cucumber)	1 1/2 cups	375 mL
Sliced green onion	1/2 cup	125 mL
Coarsely grated carrot	1/2 cup	125 mL
Large red pepper, diced	1	1

Bring first 4 ingredients to a boil in medium saucepan. Stir in rice. Reduce heat. Cover. Simmer for 15 to 20 minutes until water is absorbed and rice is cooked. Stir in rice wine. Cool to room temperature. Makes about 8 cups (2 L) rice mixture.

Line 9 x 13 inch (22 x 33 cm) pan with plastic wrap. Arrange thin even layer of lemon slices in bottom of pan. Sprinkle with capers. Cover 1/2 of pan with smoked salmon and 1/2 with shrimp. Using wet hands, pack about 2 1/2 cups (625 mL) rice mixture in an even layer on top. Lay 2 sheets of nori, trimmed to fit in single layer, on rice.

Cover nori with cucumber and green onion. Pack 2 1/2 cups (625 mL) rice on top. Layer carrot and red pepper over rice. Cover with remaining rice. Lay 2 sheets of nori, trimmed to fit in single layer, on rice. Cover with plastic wrap directly on surface.

Set another 9 x 13 inch (22 x 33 cm) pan on sushi and press down firmly to compress layers evenly. Chill for 2 hours. Remove top plastic wrap. Invert sushi onto cutting surface. Remove remaining plastic wrap. Use sharp, wet, clean knife for each cut. Makes about sixty 1 1/2 inch (3.8 cm) squares.

1 square: 40 Calories; 0.2 g Total Fat (trace Sat., 7.6 mg Cholesterol); 85 mg Sodium; 2 g Protein; 8 g Carbohydrate; trace Dietary Fibre

CHOICES: 1/2 Grains & Starches

Pictured on page 18.

Stuffed Grapevine Leaves

The fragrance while they're baking will make you very impatient to taste them! These work well served warm as an appetizer. Serve with Fresh Yogurt Sauce, page 21.

Chopped onion	1 cup	250 mL
Garlic cloves, minced	2	2
Olive oil	2 tsp.	10 mL
Brown rice	1 1/3 cups	325 mL
Medium tomato, chopped	1	1
Water	2 3/4 cups	675 mL
Chicken bouillon powder	1 tsp.	5 mL
Freshly ground pepper, sprinkle		
Chopped fresh parsley	2 tbsp.	30 mL
Raisins, chopped	1/4 cup	60 mL
Pine nuts, toasted and chopped (see Tip, page 111)	1/4 cup	60 mL
Ground cinnamon	1/4 tsp.	1 mL
Jar of grapevine leaves, drained	17 oz.	473 mL
Water	1/2 cup	125 mL
Olive oil	1 tbsp.	15 mL
Lemon juice	2 tbsp.	30 mL

Sauté onion and garlic in olive oil in large non-stick frying pan until onion is soft. Add rice. Cook until rice is toasted. Turn into large saucepan.

Stir in next 8 ingredients. Bring to a boil. Cover. Cook for about 40 minutes until rice is tender. Makes 4 1/2 cups (1.1 L).

Prepare vine leaves by pinching off any stem ends. Using larger leaves, place about 2 rounded tablespoons (30 mL) filling on underside of leaf, near stem end. Roll up, tucking in sides to enclose filling. Repeat until rice mixture is used up. Use any leftover vine leaves to line greased 3 quart (3 L) casserole. Place rolls seam side down and very close to each other in 2 layers.

Combine remaining 3 ingredients in small cup. Drizzle over rolls. Cover tightly. Bake in 325°F (160°C) oven for 1 1/2 hours until leaves are very tender and all liquid is absorbed. Makes 28 appetizers.

1 appetizer: 60 Calories; 2 g Total Fat (0.3 g Sat., trace Cholesterol); 76 mg Sodium; 2 g Protein; 10 g Carbohydrate; 1 g Dietary Fibre

CHOICES: 1/2 Grains & Starches; 1/2 Fats

Pictured on page 18.

Hummus

Serve spread on torn fresh pita or as a thick dip for vegetables.

Garlic cloves	2	2
Toasted sesame seeds (see Tip, page 111)	4 tbsp.	60 mL
Ground cumin	1/4 tsp.	1 mL
Lemon pepper	1/4 tsp.	1 mL
Lemon juice	2 tbsp.	30 mL
Can of chick peas (garbanzo beans), drained, liquid reserved	19 oz.	540 mL
Reserved chick pea liquid, approximately	7 tbsp.	115 mL

Process garlic cloves, 3 tbsp. (50 mL) sesame seeds, cumin and lemon pepper in blender on high until garlic and sesame seeds are smooth. Add enough lemon juice to make thick paste.

Add chick peas and 3 tbsp. (50 mL) chick pea liquid. Blend with pulsing motion, scraping down sides as necessary, until mixture is puréed. Add approximately 4 tbsp. (60 mL) liquid from chick peas to thin dip to desired consistency. Turn into serving bowl. Sprinkle remaining 1 tbsp. (15 mL) sesame seeds on top. Makes 2 cups (500 mL).

2 tbsp. (30 mL): 54 Calories; 1.5 g Total Fat (0.1 g Sat., 0 mg Cholesterol); 99 mg Sodium; 2 g Protein; 8 g Carbohydrate; 2 g Dietary Fibre

CHOICES: 1/2 Grains & Starches

Sangria Refresher

Garnish this fruity punch with slices of orange and lime.

Medium lime, very thinly sliced, seeded	1	1
Medium lemon, very thinly sliced, seeded	1	1
Medium oranges, very thinly sliced, seeded	2	2
Chopped fresh mint leaves (optional)	1/4 cup	60 mL
Red grape juice	1 qt.	1 L
Sugar-free ginger ale	1 qt.	1 L

Place first 4 ingredients in 2 quart (2 L) pitcher. Pour in grape juice. Chill for several hours or overnight to blend flavours.

Strain juice into large pitcher. Add ginger ale to taste. Makes 8 cups (2 L).

1/2 cup (125 mL): 48 Calories; 0.1 g Total Fat (trace Sat., 0 mg Cholesterol); 6 mg Sodium; trace Protein; 12 g Carbohydrate; trace Dietary Fibre

CHOICES: 1 Fruits

Lemonberry Smoothie

A very refreshing snack. Sip it through a straw and maybe it will last longer!

Non-fat vanilla yogurt	1 cup	250 mL
Skim milk	1/4 cup	60 mL
Frozen concentrated lemonade	3 tbsp.	50 mL
Icing (confectioner's) sugar	2 tsp.	10 mL
(or sugar substitute, such		
as Sugar Twin, to taste)		
Frozen large whole strawberries	6	6

Place first 4 ingredients in blender. Process on high, adding strawberries, 1 at a time, through lid until thick. Process, scraping down sides as necessary, until smooth. Makes 2 1/2 cups (625 mL).

3/4 cup (175 mL): 110 Calories; 0.2 g Total Fat (0.1 g Sat., 1.8 mg Cholesterol); 67 mg Sodium; 5 g Protein; 23 g Carbohydrate; 1 g Dietary Fibre

CHOICES: 1 Fruits; 1/2 Milk & Alternatives

Pictured on page 71.

Piña Colada Smoothie

Has the colour, flavour and texture of the real thing. Garnish with a slice of starfruit.

Can of crushed pineapple, with juice, chilled	14 oz.	398 mL
Coconut flavouring	1/2 tsp.	2 mL
Skim milk powder	2 tbsp.	30 mL
Non-fat vanilla yogurt	1 cup	250 mL
Ice cubes	6	6

Place first 4 ingredients in blender. Process on high, adding ice cubes, 1 at a time, through lid. As mixture becomes thick, use pulsing motion, scraping down sides occasionally, until smooth. Makes 4 cups (1 L).

3/4 cup (175 mL): 82 Calories; 0.1 g Total Fat (0.1 g Sat., 1.5 mg Cholesterol); 51 mg Sodium; 4 g Protein; 17 g Carbohydrate; 1 g Dietary Fibre

CHOICES: 1 Fruits

Pictured on page 17.

Pink Grapefruit Refresher

So refreshing! It will leave you wanting more. To serve as palate cleanser between courses, scrape from pan with an ice cream scoop and serve 3 balls per person in a tall glass.

Zest and juice from 3 medium oranges		
Zest and juice from 1 medium lemon		
Liquid honey	3 tbsp.	50 mL
Orange liqueur (optional)	1/4 cup	60 mL
Water	1/4 cup	60 mL
Large pink grapefruits	5	5
Sugar-free lemon-lime soft drink	3 cups	750 mL
Orange liqueur	1/4 cup	60 mL
Sugar-free lemon-lime soft drink, to taste		

Remove zest from oranges and lemon with vegetable peeler. Cut into long, thin slivers. Place in small saucepan. Add both juices and next 3 ingredients. Bring to a boil. Reduce heat to medium. Boil for 25 minutes until mixture is thickened and syrupy. Strain. Discard zest and pulp. Reserve syrup.

Halve and section grapefruits, discarding any seeds. Place sections in 9 × 13 inch (22 × 33 cm) glass baking pan. Scrape any remaining fruit from peel. Squeeze each half gently to drain any juices into pan. Add reserved syrup, soft drink and second amount of liqueur. Stir. Cover. Freeze for 2 hours. Break up with fork. Process in food processor or blender until smooth. Freeze. Makes 9 1/4 cups (2.3 L).

To serve, scoop about 1/2 cup (125 mL) into tall glass and fill with sugar-free lemon-lime soft drink.

1/2 cup (125 mL) without soft drink: 53 Calories; 0.1 g Total Fat (trace Sat., 0 mg Cholesterol); 3 mg Sodium; 1 g Protein; 12 g Carbohydrate; trace Dietary Fibre

CHOICES: 1/2 Fruits

Paré Pointer
A robot's favourite party snack is assorted nuts.

Cloverleaf Honey Rolls

Good, wholesome buns.

Skim milk	1 1/3 cups	325 mL
Hard margarine	1/3 cup	75 mL
Liquid honey	1/4 cup	60 mL
Salt	1 tsp.	5 mL
Whole wheat flour	2 cups	500 mL
All-purpose flour	1 cup	250 mL
Packages of instant yeast (1/4 oz., 8 g, each), or 4 1/2 tsp., (22 mL), bulk	2	2
Frozen egg product, thawed (see Note)	6 tbsp.	100 mL
All-purpose flour	2 cups	500 mL

Heat first 4 ingredients in small saucepan until margarine is melted and mixture is very warm but not hot.

Combine first 3 ingredients in large bowl. Add wet ingredients. Beat well. Add egg product. Beat.

Add all-purpose flour, 1 cup (250 mL) at a time. Work in by mixing and kneading until soft dough is formed. Turn out and knead on floured surface for 5 to 10 minutes until dough is smooth and elastic. Place in greased bowl, turning once to coat top. Cover with tea towel. Let rise in oven with light on and door closed for 1 hour until doubled in size. Punch down. Divide dough into 4 equal portions. Work with 1 portion at a time, keeping remainder covered. Shape into long roll. Cut into 9 pieces. Cut piece into 3 smaller pieces. Roll into small balls. Place 3 balls in each greased muffin cup. Repeat with remaining portions. Cover with tea towel. Let rise in oven with light on and door closed for 60 minutes until doubled in size. Bake in 400°F (205°C) oven for 10 minutes until golden brown. Makes 3 dozen rolls.

1 roll: 94 Calories; 2.1 g Total Fat (0.4 g Sat., 0.2 mg Cholesterol); 109 mg Sodium; 3 g Protein; 16 g Carbohydrate; 1 g Dietary Fibre

CHOICES: 1 Grains & Starches; 1/2 Fats

Note: 4 tbsp. (50 mL) = 1 large egg

 tip Sugar in breads acts as food for the yeast to help produce carbon dioxide, which makes the dough rise. Sugar is also used for flavour and helps the crust brown. Honey or molasses may also be used in the recipe for the same effects.

Grain Bread

This loaf is very high in fibre but still light in texture.

Large eggs	2	2
Brown sugar, packed	1/4 cup	60 mL
Fancy (mild) molasses	2 tbsp.	30 mL
Canola oil	1/2 cup	125 mL
1% buttermilk	1 qt.	1 L
Rolled oats (not instant)	1 1/2 cups	375 mL
Light rye flour	1 cup	250 mL
Natural oat bran	1/2 cup	125 mL
Packages of instant yeast (1/4 oz., 8 g, each) or 4 1/2 tsp. (22 mL) bulk	2	2
Whole wheat flour	6 1/4 cups	1.5 L

Beat first 4 ingredients in large bowl.

Heat buttermilk in medium saucepan until very warm, but not hot. Whisk or beat into egg mixture until well-blended. Mixture should still be very warm.

Combine next 4 ingredients in small bowl. Mix into buttermilk mixture until smooth. Let stand for 15 minutes.

Work or knead in enough whole wheat flour to make a sticky dough that keeps its form. Shape into 2 loaves. Place in greased 9 × 5 × 3 inch (22 × 12.5 × 7.5 cm) bread pan. Punch dough to fill in corners. Cover with greased waxed paper. Let rise in oven with door closed and light on for about 30 minutes until doubled in size. Bake in 350°F (175°C) oven for 40 minutes until hollow-sounding when tapped. Makes 2 loaves, for a total of 24 slices.

1 slice: 236 Calories; 6.8 g Total Fat (0.9 g Sat., 19.5 mg Cholesterol); 54 mg Sodium; 8 g Protein; 38 g Carbohydrate; 6 g Dietary Fibre

CHOICES: 2 Grains & Starches; 1 Fats

Pictured on page 35.

GRAIN BUNS: Shape dough into 24 buns. Place in greased 9 × 13 inch (22 × 33 cm) pan. Cover with greased waxed paper. Let rise in oven with light on and door closed for approximately 1 hour until doubled in size. Bake in 350°F (175°C) oven for 20 minutes until hollow-sounding when tapped. Makes 24 buns.

Breads & Muffins

Honey Wheat Bread

A slice of this bread is all you need for breakfast.

Very hot water	1 cup	250 mL
Liquid honey	1/4 cup	60 mL
Canola oil	2 tbsp.	30 mL
Salt	1 tsp.	5 mL
Large egg, fork-beaten	1	1
All-purpose flour	2 cups	500 mL
Package of instant yeast (or 2 1/4 tsp., 11 mL, bulk)	1/4 oz.	8 g
Whole wheat flour	1 1/4 cups	300 mL
Chopped mixed dried fruit (or raisins)	1/2 cup	125 mL

Combine first 4 ingredients in small bowl.

Put egg into large bowl. Slowly add hot water mixture, whisking until frothy.

Combine all-purpose flour and yeast in small bowl. Add to liquids. Mix well until smooth.

Slowly add whole wheat flour. Mix until soft dough is formed. Add more or less flour, as required, until soft but not too sticky.

Turn out and knead on floured surface for 10 minutes, adding dried fruit gradually, until smooth and elastic. Place in greased bowl, turning once to coat top. Cover with tea towel. Let rise in oven with light on and door closed for 1 1/2 hours until doubled in bulk. Punch down. Shape into loaf. Place in greased 9 × 5 × 3 inch (22 × 12.5 × 7.5 cm) loaf pan. Cover. Let rise until almost doubled in size. Bake in 350°F (175°C) oven for 40 to 45 minutes until hollow-sounding when tapped. If top browns too quickly, cover with foil or brown paper for last 10 minutes of baking time. Makes 1 loaf, enough for 12 slices.

1 slice: 195 Calories; 3.2 g Total Fat (0.4 g Sat., 18.0 mg Cholesterol); 234 mg Sodium; 5 g Protein; 38 g Carbohydrate; 3 g Dietary Fibre

CHOICES: 2 Grains & Starches; 1/2 Other Choices; 1/2 Fats

Pictured on page 35.

 To test the yeast for freshness, sprinkle some over warm water that has a little sugar in it. If the solution foams and bubbles, it's still active. If not, replace with new yeast.

Cinnaraisin Nut Bread

Good grain and nut flavour in these dark loaves.

Large egg	1	1
Canola oil	1 tbsp.	15 mL
Brown sugar, packed	1/2 cup	125 mL
Salt	1 tsp.	5 mL
Ground cinnamon	1 tsp.	5 mL
Skim milk	2 cups	500 mL
Package of instant yeast (or 2 1/4 tsp., 11 mL, bulk)	1/4 oz.	8 g
Whole wheat flour	1 cup	250 mL
Natural oat bran	1/2 cup	125 mL
Finely chopped toasted pecans (see Tip, page 111)	2/3 cup	150 mL
Raisins	1 cup	250 mL
All-purpose flour	3 3/4 cups	925 mL

Whisk first 5 ingredients together in small bowl.

Heat milk in small saucepan until very warm. Whisk into egg mixture.

Combine next 4 ingredients in large bowl. Add milk mixture. Whisk until smooth. Stir in raisins. Slowly work in enough all-purpose flour until dough leaves sides of bowl and is no longer sticky. Turn out and knead on lightly floured surface for about 5 minutes until smooth and elastic. Place dough in greased bowl, turning once to coat top. Cover with tea towel. Let rise in oven with light on and door closed for about 1 hour until doubled in bulk. Punch down. Knead 8 to 10 times to remove air bubbles. Shape into 2 loaves. Place in 2 greased 9 x 5 x 3 inch (22 x 12.5 x 7.5 cm) loaf pans. Cover. Let rise until doubled in size. Bake in 375°F (190°C) oven for 35 to 40 minutes until hollow-sounding when tapped. Makes 2 loaves, for a total of 24 slices.

1 slice: 176 Calories; 3.7 g Total Fat (0.4 g Sat., 9.4 mg Cholesterol); 130 mg Sodium; 5 g Protein; 33 g Carbohydrate; 2 g Dietary Fibre

CHOICES: 1 1/2 Grains & Starches; 1/2 Fats

Pictured on page 35.

Cranberry Streusel Muffins

Use orange pulp in the juice measurement for added flavour.
Moist, tender and pretty — besides being very, very good!

All-purpose flour	2 cups	500 mL
Granulated sugar	1/2 cup	125 mL
Baking powder	1 tbsp.	15 mL
Salt	1/2 tsp.	2 mL
Egg whites (large)	4	4
Hard margarine, melted	3 tbsp.	50 mL
Freshly squeezed orange juice	1 cup	250 mL
(pulp, optional)		
Grated orange zest	2 tsp.	10 mL
Chopped dried cranberries	2/3 cup	150 mL
STREUSEL TOPPING		
All-purpose flour	1/4 cup	60 mL
Brown sugar, packed	1 tbsp.	15 mL
Hard margarine	1 tbsp.	15 mL

Combine first 4 ingredients in medium bowl. Make a well in center.

Beat next 4 ingredients in small bowl until combined. Stir in cranberries. Pour into well. Stir just until moistened. Spray muffin cups with no-stick cooking spray. Fill cups 3/4 full.

Streusel Topping: Combine flour and brown sugar in small bowl. Cut in margarine until mixture is crumbly. Sprinkle 1/2 tbsp. (7 mL) over each muffin. Bake in 425°F (220°C) oven for 10 to 15 minutes until just firm. Do not overbake. Cool in pan for 5 minutes before turning out. Makes 12 muffins.

1 muffin: 190 Calories; 4 g Total Fat (0.8 g Sat., 0 mg Cholesterol); 179 mg Sodium; 4 g Protein; 35 g Carbohydrate; 2 g Dietary Fibre

CHOICES: 1 Grains & Starches; 1/2 Fruits; 1/2 Other Choices; 1 Fats

Pictured on page 35.

 tip The recipes in this cookbook use large eggs (when stated in the ingredients). If extra large eggs are used in breads, the liquid content will be higher which will cause the texture to be heavier; the extra liquid in cakes may cause them to fall when cooled.

Chili 'N' Cheese Corn Muffins

So good with soup. Chilies and chili powder give a spicy aftertaste.

Yellow cornmeal	3/4 cup	175 mL
1% buttermilk	1 cup	250 mL
Large eggs, fork-beaten	2	2
Can of diced green chilies, with liquid	4 oz.	113 g
Canola oil	1 1/2 tbsp.	25 mL
All-purpose flour	1 1/2 cups	375 mL
Baking powder	1 tbsp.	15 mL
Salt	1/2 tsp.	2 mL
Brown sugar, packed	2 tbsp.	30 mL
Chili powder	1/4 – 1/2 tsp.	1 – 2 mL
Grated light sharp Cheddar cheese	3/4 cup	175 mL

Combine first 5 ingredients in small bowl. Let stand for 15 minutes.

Combine remaining 6 ingredients in large bowl. Make a well in center. Pour cornmeal mixture into well. Stir just until moistened. Spray muffin cups with no-stick cooking spray. Fill cups 3/4 full. Bake in 375°F (190°C) oven for 20 minutes until wooden pick inserted in center of muffin comes out clean. Cool in pan for 5 minutes before turning out. Makes 12 muffins.

1 muffin: 166 Calories; 4.6 g Total Fat (1.5 g Sat., 41.2 mg Cholesterol); 311 mg Sodium; 6 g Protein; 24 g Carbohydrate; 1 g Dietary Fibre

CHOICES: 1 Grains & Starches; 1/2 Meat & Alternatives; 1 Fats

Pictured on page 35.

Orange Date Muffins

Great orange aroma and flavour. Bits of dates and raisins give sweetness.

All-purpose flour	1 1/2 cups	375 mL
Brown sugar, packed	2 tbsp.	30 mL
Baking soda	1 tsp.	5 mL
Baking powder	1 tsp.	5 mL
Salt	1/4 tsp.	1 mL
Medium orange, with peel, cut into 8 pieces	1	1
Light raisins (optional)	1/4 cup	60 mL
Chopped dates	1/4 cup	60 mL
1% buttermilk	2/3 cup	150 mL
Canola oil	3 tbsp.	50 mL
Frozen egg product, thawed (see Note)	6 tbsp.	100 mL

(continued on next page)

Combine first 5 ingredients in medium bowl. Make a well in center.

Combine remaining 6 ingredients in blender. Process until orange, raisins and dates are well-chopped. Pour into well. Stir just until moistened. Spray muffin cups with no-stick cooking spray. Fill cups 3/4 full. Bake in 400°F (205°C) oven for 18 to 20 minutes until wooden pick inserted in center of muffin comes out clean. Cool in pan for 5 minutes before turning out. Makes 12 muffins.

1 muffin: 135 Calories; 3.9 g Total Fat (0.4 g Sat., 0.5 mg Cholesterol); 209 mg Sodium; 4 g Protein; 23 g Carbohydrate; 2 g Dietary Fibre

CHOICES: 1 Grains & Starches; 1/2 Fruits; 1 Fats

Pictured on page 35.

Note: 4 tbsp. (50 mL) = 1 large egg

Carrot Pineapple Muffins

A very moist muffin with a definite pineapple flavour.

All-purpose flour	1 1/3 cups	325 mL
Quick-cooking rolled oats (not instant)	1 cup	250 mL
Brown sugar, packed	1/2 cup	125 mL
Baking powder	1 1/2 tbsp.	25 mL
Ground cinnamon	1/2 tsp.	2 mL
Salt	1/4 tsp.	1 mL
Ground nutmeg	1/8 tsp.	0.5 mL
Frozen egg product, thawed (see Note)	1/4 cup	60 mL
Canola oil	1/4 cup	60 mL
Non-fat vanilla yogurt	1/2 cup	125 mL
Canned crushed pineapple, well-drained	1 cup	250 mL
Grated carrot	1/2 cup	125 mL

Combine first 7 ingredients in large bowl. Make a well in center.

Combine remaining 5 ingredients in small bowl. Pour into well. Stir just until moistened. Spray muffin cups with no-stick cooking spray. Fill cups 3/4 full. Bake in 400°F (205°C) oven for 20 minutes until wooden pick inserted in center of muffin comes out clean. Cool in pan for 5 minutes before turning out. Makes 12 muffins.

1 muffin: 182 Calories; 5.6 g Total Fat (0.5 g Sat., 0.2 mg Cholesterol); 86 mg Sodium; 4 g Protein; 30 g Carbohydrate; 2 g Dietary Fibre

CHOICES: 1 Grains & Starches; 1/2 Other Choices; 1 Fats

Note: 4 tbsp. (50 mL) = 1 large egg

Cornbread Muffins

The bits of corn give off a touch of sweetness. Makes a big batch.
These freeze well and can be warmed for lunch.

Yellow cornmeal	1 1/2 cups	375 mL
1% buttermilk	1 1/3 cups	325 mL
All-purpose flour	3 cups	750 mL
Brown sugar, packed	1/4 cup	60 mL
Baking powder	2 tbsp.	30 mL
Salt	1 tsp.	5 mL
Frozen egg product, thawed (see Note)	1 cup	250 mL
Canola oil	1/3 cup	75 mL
Can of cream-style corn	14 oz.	398 mL

Combine cornmeal and buttermilk in medium bowl. Let stand for 15 minutes.

Combine next 4 ingredients in large bowl. Make a well in center.

Combine remaining 3 ingredients in small bowl. Add to cornmeal mixture.
Mix well. Pour into well. Stir just until moistened. Spray muffin cups with no-stick
cooking spray. Fill cups 3/4 full. Bake in 375°F (190°C) oven for 15 to 17 minutes
until wooden pick inserted in center of muffin comes out clean. Cool in pan for
5 minutes before turning out. Makes 24 muffins.

*1 muffin: 157 Calories; 3.8 g Total Fat (0.4 g Sat., 0.5 mg Cholesterol); 205 mg Sodium; 4 g Protein;
27 g Carbohydrate; 1 g Dietary Fibre*

CHOICES: 1 1/2 Grains & Starches; 1 Fats

Note: 4 tbsp. (50 mL) = 1 large egg

1. Honey Wheat Bread, page 29
2. Cinnaraisin Nut Bread, page 30
3. Grain Bread, page 28
4. Chili 'N' Cheese Corn Muffins, page 32
5. Pumpkin Raisin Muffins, page 38
6. Cranberry Streusel Muffins, page 31
7. Orange Date Muffins, page 32
8. Onion Cheese Biscuits, page 39

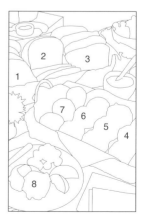

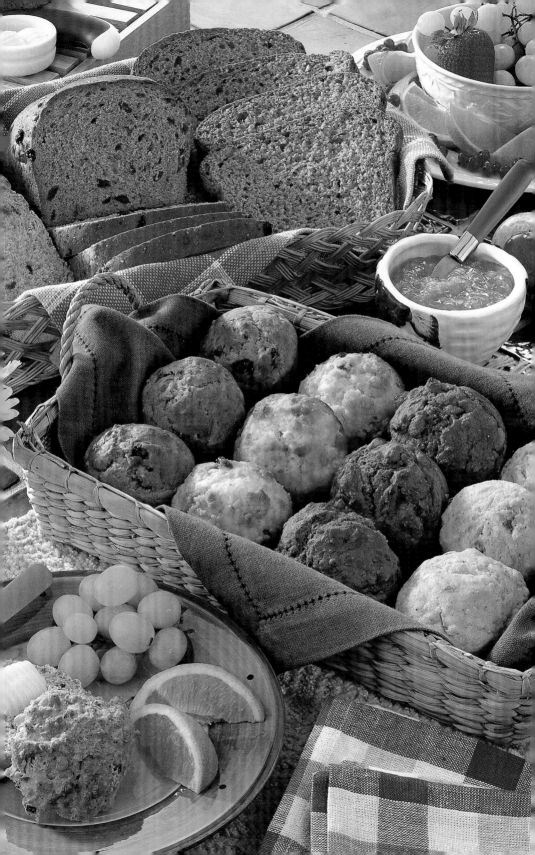

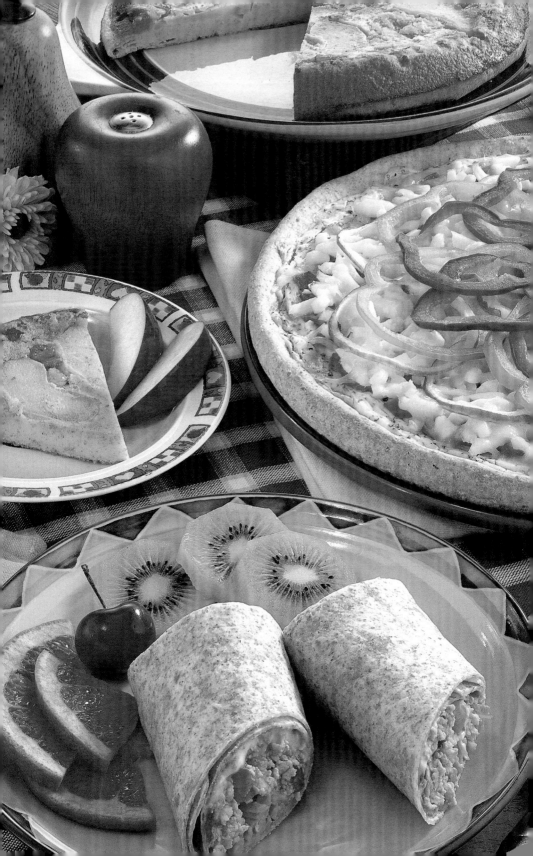

Oatmeal Apple Muffins

Nice texture with bits of apple. A good breakfast or snack.

Whole wheat flour	1 1/4 cups	300 mL
Quick-cooking rolled oats (not instant)	1 cup	250 mL
Brown sugar, packed	1/3 cup	75 mL
Baking powder	2 1/2 tsp.	12 mL
Baking soda	1/4 tsp.	1 mL
Salt	1/4 tsp.	1 mL
Ground nutmeg	1/4 tsp.	1 mL
Ground cinnamon	1/4 tsp.	1 mL
1% buttermilk	1 cup	250 mL
Large egg, fork-beaten	1	1
Canola oil	2 tbsp.	30 mL
Medium apple, peeled and diced	1	1

Combine first 8 ingredients in large bowl. Make a well in center.

Combine next 3 ingredients in small bowl. Pour into well. Add apple. Stir just until moistened. Spray muffin cups with no-stick cooking spray. Fill cups 1/2 full. Bake in 375°F (190°C) oven for 15 to 18 minutes until wooden pick inserted in center of muffin comes out clean. Cool in pan for 5 minutes before turning out. Makes 12 muffins.

1 muffin: 139 Calories; 3.7 g Total Fat (0.6 g Sat., 18.7 mg Cholesterol); 119 mg Sodium; 4 g Protein; 24 g Carbohydrate; 3 g Dietary Fibre

CHOICES: 1 Grains & Starches; 1/2 Fats

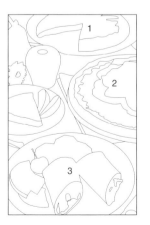

1. Apple Clafouti, page 44
2. G'Morning Pizza, page 40
3. Morning Burritos, page 45

Props courtesy of: The Bay

Pumpkin Raisin Muffins

Raisins in every bite in these spiced muffins.

All-purpose flour	1 cup	250 mL
Whole wheat flour	3/4 cup	175 mL
Natural oat bran	1/4 cup	60 mL
Brown sugar, packed	1/2 cup	125 mL
Baking soda	1 1/2 tsp.	7 mL
Baking powder	1 tsp.	5 mL
Ground cinnamon	1 tsp.	5 mL
Ground nutmeg	1/2 tsp.	2 mL
Ground allspice	1/4 tsp.	1 mL
Salt	1/4 tsp.	1 mL
Can of pumpkin (without spices)	14 oz.	398 mL
Large egg, fork-beaten	1	1
Skim milk	1 cup	250 mL
Canola oil	2 tbsp.	30 mL
Grated lemon zest	1 tsp.	5 mL
Raisins	1 cup	250 mL

Combine first 10 ingredients in large bowl. Make a well in center.

Beat together next 5 ingredients in medium bowl until smooth. Pour into well. Stir until barely combined Add raisins. Stir just until moistened. Spray muffin cups with no-stick cooking spray. Fill cups 3/4 full. Bake in 400°F (205°C) oven for 20 minutes until wooden pick inserted in center of muffin comes out clean. Cool in pan for 5 minutes before turning out. Makes 12 muffins.

1 muffin: 194 Calories; 3.4 g Total Fat (0.5 g Sat., 18.4 mg Cholesterol); 196 mg Sodium; 5 g Protein; 39 g Carbohydrate; 3 g Dietary Fibre

CHOICES: 1 Grains & Starches; 1/2 Fruits; 1/2 Vegetable; 1/2 Other Choices; 1 Fats

Pictured on page 35.

Onion Cheese Biscuits

Delicious warm with soup or salad, or just some fresh fruit.

All-purpose flour	1 cup	250 mL
Whole wheat flour	1 cup	250 mL
Baking powder	2 tsp.	10 mL
Baking soda	1/2 tsp.	2 mL
Grated light sharp Cheddar cheese	1 cup	250 mL
Dill weed	1 tsp.	5 mL
Salt	1/4 tsp.	1 mL
Freshly ground pepper	1/8 tsp.	0.5 mL
Non-fat plain yogurt	3/4 cup	175 mL
Skim milk	1/2 cup	125 mL
Canola oil	2 tbsp.	30 mL
Green onions, chopped	4	4

Combine first 8 ingredients in large bowl.

Combine remaining 4 ingredients in small bowl. Add to flour mixture. Stir just until moistened. Drop by large spoonfuls onto greased baking sheet. Bake in center of 400°F (205°C) oven for 12 to 15 minutes until golden brown. Makes 12 biscuits.

1 biscuit: 140 Calories; 4.6 g Total Fat (1.5 g Sat., 6.5 mg Cholesterol); 199 mg Sodium; 6 g Protein; 18 g Carbohydrate; 2 g Dietary Fibre

CHOICES: 1 Grains & Starches; 1/2 Fats

Pictured on page 35.

Paré Pointer

What's the difference between the law and a glacier?
The law is justice, while a glacier is just ice.

G' Morning Pizza

A nice brunch for the whole family.

All-purpose flour	1 cup	250 mL
Whole wheat flour	1/2 cup	125 mL
Instant yeast	1 1/2 tsp.	7 mL
Grated light Parmesan cheese	1 tbsp.	15 mL
Dried sweet basil	1/2 tsp.	2 mL
Dried whole oregano	1/4 tsp.	1 mL
Salt	1/2 tsp.	2 mL
Very warm water	2/3 cup	150 mL
Canola oil	2 tsp.	10 mL
Large hard-boiled eggs, peeled	6	6
Light cream cheese	4 oz.	125 g
Parsley flakes	1/2 tsp.	2 mL
Dried sweet basil	1/2 tsp.	2 mL
Garlic powder	1/16 tsp.	0.5 mL
Fat-free ham slices, diced	2/3 cup	150 mL
Grated part-skim mozzarella cheese	1 cup	250 mL
Thinly sliced red onion	1/2 cup	125 mL
Thinly sliced green and red peppers	2/3 cup	150 mL
Dried sweet basil, sprinkle (optional)		
Dried whole oregano, sprinkle (optional)		

Combine first 7 ingredients in food processor or medium bowl.

Combine water and canola oil in small bowl. Add through chute while processing until dough forms ball (or if mixing in bowl, stir in water and canola oil until dough leaves sides of bowl). Turn out and knead for 3 to 4 minutes until smooth. Cover. Let stand for 15 minutes. Press lightly in greased 12 inch (30 cm) pizza pan. Form raised rim around edge. Bake in 425°F (220°C) oven for 8 minutes, poking any bubbles with fork.

Discard 4 yolks. Chop remaining egg whites and 2 whole eggs.

Combine next 4 ingredients in small bowl. Spread onto hot crust. Layer with eggs and next 4 ingredients, in order. Sprinkle with basil and oregano. Bake in center of 425°F (220°C) oven for 8 to 10 minutes until cheese is melted and crust is browned. Cuts into 8 wedges.

1 wedge: 215 Calories; 8 g Total Fat (2.9 g Sat., 66.4 mg Cholesterol); 648 mg Sodium; 13 g Protein; 23 g Carbohydrate; 2 g Dietary Fibre

CHOICES: 1 Grains & Starches; 1 Meat & Alternatives; 1 Fats

Pictured on page 36.

Ham 'N' Apple Strata

Golden crisp topping with layers of ham, apple and bread.

Whole wheat bread slices, crusts removed	8	8
Fat-free ham slices	4 1/2 oz.	125 g
Large apple, cored and cut into thin wedges	1	1
Grated light sharp Cheddar cheese	1/2 cup	125 mL
Carton of frozen egg product, thawed (see Note)	8 oz.	227 mL
Egg whites (large)	4	4
Skim evaporated milk	1 cup	250 mL
Water	1/2 cup	125 mL
Seasoned salt	1/2 tsp.	2 mL
Hot pepper sauce	1/4 tsp.	1 mL
Corn flakes cereal	1 cup	250 mL
Margarine, melted	1 tbsp.	15 mL
Grated light sharp Cheddar cheese	1/2 cup	125 mL

Place 4 slices of bread in greased shallow 2 quart (2 L) casserole or 9 x 9 inch (22 x 22 cm) pan. Layer bread with next 3 ingredients, in order. Cover with remaining 4 bread slices.

Beat next 6 ingredients together. Slowly pour onto bread slices. Cover tightly with plastic wrap. Chill overnight.

Crush cereal in small bowl. Add margarine and second amount of cheese. Stir. Sprinkle over strata. Bake, uncovered, in 350°F (175°C) oven for 50 to 55 minutes until set and top is golden brown. Let stand for 15 minutes before cutting. Cuts into 4 pieces.

1 piece: 412 Calories; 10.8 g Total Fat (4.7 g Sat., 22 mg Cholesterol); 1367 mg Sodium; 32 g Protein; 49 g Carbohydrate; 4 g Dietary Fibre

CHOICES: 2 Grains & Starches; 1/2 Milk & Alternatives; 3 Meat & Alternatives; 1/2 Fats

Note: 4 tbsp. (50 mL) = 1 large egg

 Grated light sharp Cheddar cheese provides a big hit of flavour without all the fat of regular Cheddar cheese. Try other light cheeses on the market to find great taste that's not heavy on fat grams.

Baked Omelette Puff

Layered look when cut. Removes easily in wedges.

Margarine	1 tsp.	5 mL
Finely diced red pepper	1/4 cup	60 mL
Sliced green onion	1/4 cup	60 mL
Diced zucchini, with peel	1/2 cup	125 mL
Sliced fresh mushrooms	1/2 cup	125 mL
Salt	1/2 tsp.	2 mL
Freshly ground pepper, generous sprinkle		
Egg yolks (large)	4	4
Egg whites (large)	8	8
Grated light sharp Cheddar cheese	1/2 cup	125 mL
Paprika, sprinkle		

Heat margarine in medium non-stick frying pan until bubbling. Add next 4 ingredients. Stir. Cook on medium-high until liquid has evaporated. Stir in salt and pepper. Cool to room temperature.

Beat egg yolks in small bowl until thick and lemon-coloured. Stir into vegetables.

Beat egg whites with clean beaters in large bowl until soft peaks form. Gently fold in vegetable mixture and cheese. Pour into well-greased 10 inch (25 cm) glass pie plate or 2 quart (2 L) casserole. Sprinkle with paprika. Bake in 350°F (175°C) oven for about 25 minutes until knife inserted in center comes out clean. Cuts into 8 wedges.

1 wedge: 77 Calories; 4.5 g Total Fat (2.4 g Sat., 149.6 mg Cholesterol); 283 mg Sodium; 7 g Protein; 2 g Carbohydrate; trace Dietary Fibre

CHOICES: 1 Meat & Alternatives; 1 Fats

Hot Wheat Berry Pudding

Satisfies your chewy cravings with nice sweetness.

Wheat berries (unprocessed wheat kernels)	1 1/4 cups	300 mL
Water	4 1/4 cups	1 L
Mixed dried fruit, with raisins, chopped if large	1 cup	250 mL
Long thread (or flake) coconut	1/3 cup	75 mL
Coarsely chopped almonds	1/4 cup	60 mL
Brown sugar, packed	3 tbsp.	50 mL
Non-fat vanilla yogurt	2 cups	500 mL

(continued on next page)

Cook wheat berries in water in large saucepan for 1 1/4 hours until tender but still quite chewy.

Stir in next 4 ingredients. Let stand for 5 minutes. Makes 5 cups (1.25 L) cooked wheat mixture. Add 1/4 cup (60 mL) yogurt to individual servings. Stir. Serves 8.

1 serving: 254 Calories; 5.4 g Total Fat (2.6 g Sat., 1.2 mg Cholesterol); 53 mg Sodium; 9 g Protein; 47 g Carbohydrate; 5 g Dietary Fibre

CHOICES: 1 Grains & Starches; 1 Fruits; 1/2 Milk & Alternatives; 1 Fats

Buttermilk Pancakes

Serve with Blueberry Sauce or Danish Cream Topping, page 46, for a special treat.

Whole wheat flour	3/4 cup	175 mL
All-purpose flour	3/4 cup	175 mL
Brown sugar, packed	2 tbsp.	30 mL
Baking powder	1 tbsp.	15 mL
Baking soda	1/2 tsp.	2 mL
Salt	1/4 tsp.	1 mL
1% buttermilk	1 1/2 cups	375 mL
Egg yolks (large)	2	2
Canola oil	3 tbsp.	50 mL
Egg whites (large)	2	2

Combine first 6 ingredients in medium bowl.

Whisk next 3 ingredients in small bowl. Add to dry ingredients. Stir just until moistened. Batter will be lumpy.

Beat egg whites in small bowl until stiff. Fold into batter. Pour batter into non-stick frying pan. Cook on medium-low for 3 to 5 minutes per side until golden brown. Makes 12 pancakes.

1 pancake: 123 Calories; 4.8 g Total Fat (0.7 g Sat., 37.1 mg Cholesterol); 164 mg Sodium; 4 g Protein; 16 g Carbohydrate; 1 g Dietary Fibre

CHOICES: 1 Grains & Starches; 1/2 Fats

Apple Clafouti

Custard consistency with crunchy apples.

Large cooking apple (such as McIntosh), peeled, cored and cut into thin wedges	1	1
Light raisins	1/4 cup	60 mL
Brown sugar, packed	2 tbsp.	30 mL
Ground cinnamon	1/4 tsp.	1 mL
Skim milk	1 1/4 cups	300 mL
Canola oil	1 tbsp.	15 mL
Frozen egg product, thawed (see Note)	1/2 cup	125 mL
Vanilla	1 tsp.	5 mL
Whole wheat flour	1/3 cup	75 mL
All-purpose flour	1/3 cup	75 mL
Granulated sugar	1/4 cup	60 mL
Ground cinnamon	1/4 tsp.	1 mL

Overlap apple wedges in circle in bottom of well-greased 9 inch (22 cm) glass pie plate. Sprinkle with next 3 ingredients.

Beat next 4 ingredients in medium bowl. Add remaining 4 ingredients. Beat until smooth. Pour batter evenly over apple. Bake in center of 375°F (190°C) oven for 40 minutes until set and golden brown. Cuts into 6 wedges.

1 wedge: 187 Calories; 2.8 g Total Fat (0.3 g Sat., 1.0 mg Cholesterol); 71 mg Sodium; 6 g Protein; 36 g Carbohydrate; 2 g Dietary Fibre

CHOICES: 1 Grains & Starches; 1/2 Fruits; 1/2 Other Choices; 1/2 Meat & Alternatives

Pictured on page 36.

Note: 4 tbsp. (50 mL) = 1 large egg

tip   To plump raisins or other dried fruit, cover with boiling water. Let stand for one minute, then drain.

Morning Burritos

Makes a great breakfast for the whole family. Serve with fresh fruit.

Chopped green onion	1/4 cup	60 mL
Margarine	2 tsp.	10 mL
Frozen egg product, thawed (see Note)	1 cup	250 mL
Chili powder	1/4 tsp.	1 mL
Salt	1/4 tsp.	1 mL
Chopped pickled hot peppers	2 tbsp.	30 mL
Grated light sharp Cheddar cheese	3/4 cup	175 mL
Whole wheat flour tortillas (10 inch, 25 cm, size), warmed	4	4
Salsa (optional)	2 tbsp.	30 mL
Light sour cream (optional)	2 tbsp.	30 mL

Sauté green onion in margarine in large non-stick frying pan for 30 seconds. Pour in egg product. Sprinkle with chili powder and salt. Heat, stirring occasionally, on medium until egg starts to set. Add peppers. Heat until egg is cooked.

Divide and sprinkle cheese over tortillas. Place 1/4 of egg mixture in line down center of each tortilla over cheese. Top egg mixture with salsa and sour cream. Roll tortillas mixture, tucking in sides, to enclose filling. Cut in half to serve. Makes 4 burritos.

1 burrito: 284 Calories; 7.6 g Total Fat (3.4 g Sat., 13.5 mg Cholesterol); 705 mg Sodium; 18 g Protein; 35 g Carbohydrate; 1 g Dietary Fibre

CHOICES: 2 Grains & Starches; 2 Meat & Alternatives; 1/2 Fats

Pictured on page 36.

Note: 4 tbsp. (50 mL) = 1 large egg

Paré Pointer
You can always tell a dogwood tree by its bark.

Blueberry Sauce

This is very good with Buttermilk Pancakes, page 43.

Fresh (or frozen, thawed) blueberries	3 cups	750 mL
Unsweetened apple juice	1/2 cup	125 mL
Cornstarch	4 tsp.	20 mL
Cold water	2 tbsp.	30 mL
Lemon juice	1 tsp.	5 mL
Vanilla	1/2 tsp.	2 mL
Sugar substitute (such as Sugar Twin)	2 tbsp.	30 mL

Place blueberries and apple juice in medium saucepan. Simmer on medium for about 4 to 8 minutes until blueberries start to break apart and are soft.

Combine cornstarch with water in small dish. Stir into blueberries. Bring to a boil. Boil for about 2 minutes on low until clear and thickened. Remove from heat.

Stir in remaining 3 ingredients. Serve warm or at room temperature. Makes 2 cups (500 mL).

1/4 cup (60 mL): 46 Calories; 0.2 g Total Fat (0 g Sat., 0 mg Cholesterol); 4 mg Sodium; trace Protein; 11 g Carbohydrate; 2 g Dietary Fibre

CHOICES: 1/2 Fruits

Danish Cream Topping

Great on Buttermilk Pancakes, page 43, and any whole grain toast or bagel. Freezes well.

Non-fat creamed cottage cheese	2 cups	500 mL
Skim milk	2 tbsp.	30 mL
Liquid honey	1 tbsp.	15 mL
Finely grated orange zest	1/2 tsp.	2 mL
Ground cinnamon	1/4 tsp.	1 mL
Almond flavouring	1/4 tsp.	1 mL

Place all 6 ingredients in blender. Process for 2 minutes, scraping down sides as necessary, until puréed. Makes 2 cups (500 mL).

2 tbsp. (30 mL): 30 Calories; trace Total Fat (0 g Sat., trace Cholesterol); 54 mg Sodium; 5 g Protein; 2 g Carbohydrate; trace Dietary Fibre

CHOICES: 1 Meat & Alternatives

French Pastry Dessert

A bit fussy to make, but it will get rave reviews. Must sit for
24 hours for soda crackers to soften into pastry layers.

All-purpose flour	3 tbsp.	50 mL
Cornstarch	3 tbsp.	50 mL
Salt	1/4 tsp.	1 mL
Can of skim evaporated milk	13 1/2 oz.	385 mL
Skim milk	1 1/3 cups	325 mL
Sugar substitute (such as Sugar Twin)	1/3 cup	75 mL
Large egg, fork-beaten	1	1
Vanilla	2 tsp.	10 mL
Yellow food colouring (optional)		
Unsalted soda crackers	48	48
Light frozen whipped topping, thawed	4 cups	1 L
Can of sliced peaches in pear juice, drained	14 oz.	398 mL

Combine first 3 ingredients in heavy-bottomed medium saucepan. Slowly add both milks. Whisk until smooth. Heat and stir on medium until boiling and thickened.

Whisk next 3 ingredients in small bowl. Add two spoonfuls of hot milk mixture to bowl. Mix well. Add to saucepan. Whisk together. Add food colouring to make custard colour. Heat, stirring constantly, for 1 to 2 minutes until slightly thickened. Cover with plastic wrap directly on surface to prevent skin from forming. Cool to room temperature. Custard should still be runny, not set.

Line bottom of 9 × 9 inch (22 × 22 cm) pan with single layer of 16 crackers. Pour over or spoon on 1 cup (250 mL) custard in even layer. Spoon 1 1/3 cups (325 mL) whipped topping in small dabs over custard. Spread carefully. Repeat cracker, custard and topping layers 2 more times, finishing with topping. Cover dessert with plastic wrap. Chill for at least 24 hours.

Arrange peaches on surface. Cuts into 9 pieces.

1 piece: 247 Calories; 6.1 g Total Fat (4.3 g Sat., 22.6 mg Cholesterol); 272 mg Sodium; 8 g Protein; 42 g Carbohydrate; 1 g Dietary Fibre

CHOICES: 1 Grains & Starches; 1/2 Fruits; 1/2 Milk & Alternatives

Almond Cheesecake

Good cheesecake texture and flavour. The variation
with fresh fruit is delicious as well.

CRUST		
Digestive biscuit crumbs (about 8 biscuits)	1 1/4 cups	300 mL
Ground almonds	1/4 cup	60 mL
Margarine, melted	2 tbsp.	30 mL
Water	1 tbsp.	15 mL
FILLING		
Envelopes of unflavoured gelatin (1/4 oz., 7 g, each)	2	2
Skim milk	1/4 cup	60 mL
1% buttermilk	1 1/4 cups	300 mL
Light ricotta cheese	1 1/2 cups	375 mL
Sugar substitute (such as Sugar Twin)	1/4 – 1/3 cup	60 – 75 mL
Almond flavouring	1/2 tsp.	2 mL
Light frozen whipped topping, thawed	2 cups	500 mL
Sliced almonds, toasted (see Tip, page 111)	2 tbsp.	30 mL

Crust: Combine first 3 ingredients in small bowl. Add water, 1 tsp. (5 mL) at a time, until crumbs stick together when squeezed. Press firmly into greased 9 inch (22 cm) springform pan. Bake in 325°F (160°C) oven for 10 minutes. Cool.

Filling: Combine gelatin and milk in small dish. Let stand for 5 minutes. Microwave on high (100%) for 10 seconds or heat over hot water. Stir to dissolve gelatin. Let stand at room temperature until cooled slightly but still liquid (see Note).

Beat next 4 ingredients in large bowl for several minutes until light and frothy. Beat in gelatin mixture. Fold in whipped topping. Pour into crust.

Sprinkle with almonds, pressing in slightly. Cover. Chill for several hours or overnight until firm. Cuts into 10 wedges.

1 wedge: 209 Calories; 11.1 g Total Fat (5.1 g Sat., 13.3 mg Cholesterol); 213 mg Sodium;
9 g Protein; 20 g Carbohydrate; 1 g Dietary Fibre

CHOICES: 1 Grains & Starches; 1/2 Meat & Alternatives; 1 Fats

LEMON CHEESECAKE: Omit almond flavouring. Add 1/2 tsp. (2 mL) lemon flavouring. Fold 1 tsp. (5 mL) grated lemon zest into filling with whipped topping. Serve with Fresh Fruit Salad, page 67.

Note: If gelatin mixture becomes lumpy as it starts to set, warm it gently and stir until it is liquid again.

Rainbow Fruit Pizza

So pretty, so delicious and so refreshing. Uses Tangy Lemon Spread, page 60.

CRUST		
All-purpose flour	3/4 cup	175 mL
Quick-cooking rolled oats (not instant)	1/2 cup	125 mL
Brown sugar, packed	1 tbsp.	15 mL
Salt	1/8 tsp.	0.5 mL
Cold hard margarine, cut into 6 pieces	1/4 cup	60 mL
Ice water	3 tbsp.	50 mL
Tangy Lemon Spread, page 60	1 cup	250 mL
Fresh (or frozen, thawed) blueberries	1 cup	250 mL
Sliced fresh strawberries	1 cup	250 mL
Small kiwifruit, peeled and sliced	2	2
Envelope of unflavoured gelatin	1/4 oz.	7 g
Unsweetened orange juice	1/3 cup	75 mL
Liquid honey (optional)	2 tsp.	10 mL

Crust: Process first 4 ingredients in food processor or blender until oats are powdery. Add margarine. Pulse with on/off motion until crumbly.

Drizzle water, 1 tbsp. (15 mL) at a time, over dry ingredients. Pulse 4 to 5 times after each addition. Add enough water to make a ball. Roll out dough to 10 inch (25 cm) circle. Place on lightly greased baking sheet. Roll edge, making fluted design. Poke all over with fork. Chill. Bake in 450°F (230°C) oven for 12 to 15 minutes until golden brown. Cool on wire rack.

Spread crust with Tangy Lemon Spread. Arrange fruit in single layer on crust.

Soften gelatin in orange juice in small saucepan for 1 minute. Heat and stir on low until dissolved. Stir in honey. Cool to room temperature. Brush liberally on fruit. Chill well. Cuts into 10 wedges.

1 wedge: 153 Calories; 5.5 g Total Fat (1.1 g Sat., 0.3 mg Cholesterol); 107 mg Sodium; 4 g Protein; 23 g Carbohydrate; 2 g Dietary Fibre

CHOICES: 1 Grains & Starches; 1/2 Fruits; 1 Fats

Chocolate Mousse

An excellent filling for phyllo cups or meringues.

Cocoa	2 tbsp.	30 mL
Cornstarch	1 tbsp.	15 mL
All-purpose flour	1 tbsp.	15 mL
Salt	1/8 tsp.	0.5 mL
Can of skim evaporated milk	13 1/2 oz.	385 mL
Frozen egg product, thawed (see Note)	1/2 cup	125 mL
Envelope of unflavoured gelatin	1/4 oz.	7 g
Cold water	1/4 cup	60 mL
Sugar substitute (such as Sugar Twin)	1/4 cup	60 mL
Vanilla	1 tsp.	5 mL
Egg whites (large)	3	3

Light frozen whipped topping, for garnish
Shaved chocolate, for garnish

Combine first 4 ingredients in medium saucepan. Slowly whisk in evaporated milk until smooth. Heat on medium, stirring frequently, until boiling and slightly thickened. Remove from heat.

Measure egg product into small bowl. Stir in two large spoonfuls of chocolate mixture. Slowly whisk back into chocolate mixture.

Combine gelatin and water in small dish. Let stand for 5 minutes. Whisk into chocolate mixture. Heat and stir on medium for 2 to 3 minutes until slightly thickened. Do not boil. Remove from heat.

Stir in sugar substitute and vanilla. Cover with plastic wrap directly on surface to prevent skin from forming. Cool for about 30 minutes until starting to set around the edges. Beat on high speed in large bowl for several minutes until thickened and creamy.

With clean beaters, beat egg whites in medium bowl until soft peaks form. Gently fold egg whites into chocolate mixture. Cover. Chill several hours or overnight until set.

Garnish with whipped topping and chocolate. Makes 4 cups (1 L).

1/2 cup (125 mL): 70 Calories; 0.3 g Total Fat (0.1 g Sat., 1.9 mg Cholesterol); 156 mg Sodium; 8 g Protein; 9 g Carbohydrate; 1 g Dietary Fibre

CHOICES: 1/2 Meat & Alternatives

Pictured on page 53.

Note: 4 tbsp. (50 mL) = 1 large egg

Cherry Chocolate Dessert

Fluffy and pretty topping on a fudgy base. So good you won't believe it's low fat!

Brownies, page 59		
Envelope of unflavoured gelatin	1/4 oz.	7 g
Reserved cherry syrup		
Package of sugar-free cherry-flavoured gelatin (jelly powder)	1/3 oz.	11 g
Can of pitted cherries in syrup, drained, syrup reserved, chopped	14 oz.	398 mL
Non-fat spreadable cream cheese	8 oz.	225 g
Light liquid topping (such as Nutriwhip)	1 cup	250 mL
Chocolate curls, for garnish		

Bake Brownies in greased 9 inch (22 cm) springform pan. Cool in pan. Do not glaze. Do not remove sides from pan.

Sprinkle unflavoured gelatin over reserved syrup in small saucepan. Let stand for 5 minutes. Heat and stir on medium until boiling. Pour into large bowl.

Stir in jelly powder until dissolved. Stir in cherries. Whisk in cream cheese until well-blended. Chill for about 15 minutes, stirring 3 to 4 times, until syrupy and cherries stay suspended.

Beat liquid topping in large bowl until stiff peaks form. Fold into cherry mixture. Spread over Brownies to edge of pan. Chill for 4 to 5 hours until set. Remove sides from pan.

Garnish with chocolate curls. Cuts into 12 pieces.

1 piece: 246 Calories; 9 g Total Fat (1.4 g Sat., 0 mg Cholesterol); 59 mg Sodium; 5 g Protein; 40 g Carbohydrate; 3 g Dietary Fibre

CHOICES: 1/2 Grains & Starches; 1/2 Fruits; 1 1/2 Other Choices; 1/2 Meat & Alternatives; 1 1/2 Fats

Pictured on page 53.

Pineapple Nut Kuchen

This kuchen (KOO-ken) is a not-too-sweet dessert that is also great served at brunch.

All-purpose flour	1/2 cup	125 mL
Yellow cornmeal	1/2 cup	125 mL
Quick-cooking rolled oats (not instant)	1/3 cup	75 mL
Baking powder	1 tsp.	5 mL
Baking soda	1/8 tsp.	0.5 mL
Ground cinnamon	1/8 tsp.	0.5 mL
Non-fat plain yogurt	1/2 cup	125 mL
Large egg, fork-beaten	1	1
Brown sugar, packed	1/4 cup	60 mL
Margarine, melted	2 tbsp.	30 mL
Can of pineapple tidbits, well-drained	14 oz.	398 mL
Chopped pecans	2 tbsp.	30 mL
Liquid honey, warmed	2 tbsp.	30 mL

Combine first 6 ingredients in medium bowl.

Beat next 4 ingredients in small bowl. Add to dry ingredients. Stir just until moistened. Turn into greased small quiche dish or 9 inch (22 cm) glass pie plate.

Scatter pineapple and pecans over top of batter. Press lightly with palm of hand. Drizzle with honey. Bake, uncovered, in 350°F (175°C) oven for 25 minutes until wooden pick inserted in center comes out clean. Serve warm. Cuts into 8 wedges.

1 wedge: 188 Calories; 5.1 g Total Fat (0.9 g Sat., 27.2 mg Cholesterol); 79 mg Sodium; 4 g Protein; 32 g Carbohydrate; 2 g Dietary Fibre

CHOICES: 1 Grains & Starches; 1/2 Other Choices; 1 Fats

Pictured at right.

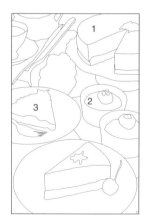

1. Cherry Chocolate Dessert, page 51
2. Chocolate Mousse, page 50
3. Pineapple Nut Kuchen, above

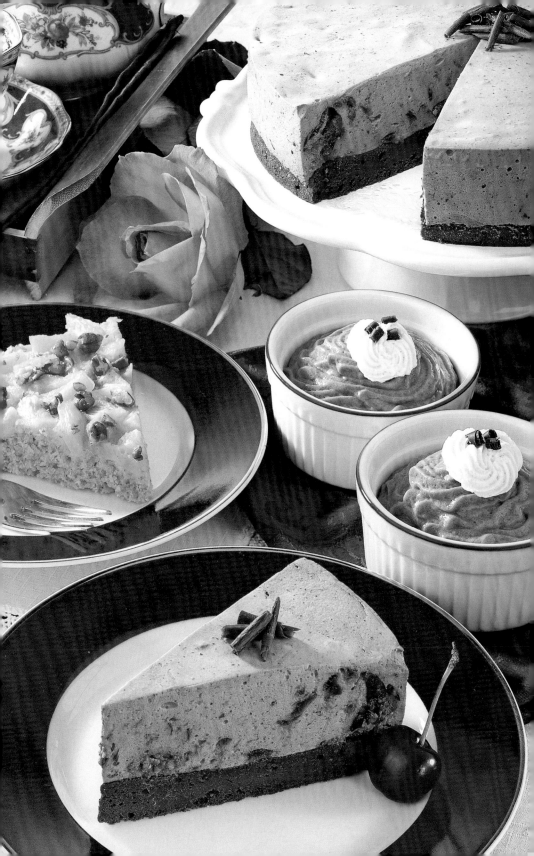

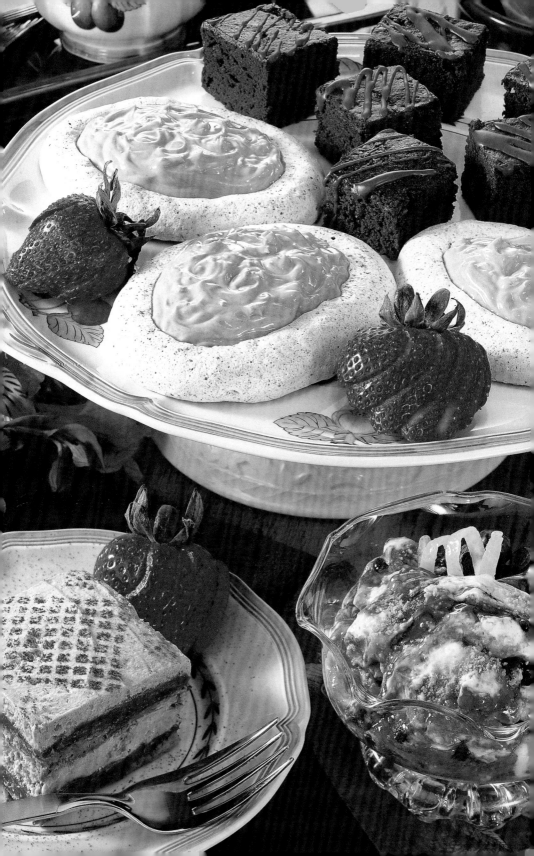

Lemon Chiffon Filling

Fluffy, light and airy—all describe this fresh-tasting filling.
Great for individual puddings or a pie.

Envelopes of unflavoured gelatin (1/4 oz., 7 g, each)	2	2
Unsweetened pineapple juice	1 cup	250 mL
Liquid honey	1 tbsp.	15 mL
Salt, pinch		
Lemon juice	3 tbsp.	50 mL
Grated lemon zest	1 tsp.	5 mL
Drops of yellow food coloring (optional)	3	3
Light frozen whipped topping	2 cups	500 mL
Non-fat lemon yogurt	1 cup	250 mL

Sprinkle gelatin over pineapple juice in medium saucepan. Let stand for 5 minutes. Heat and stir on medium until gelatin is dissolved. Stir in next 5 ingredients. Chill, stirring several times, until syrupy.

Fold whipped topping into gelatin mixture. Fold in yogurt. Pour into 8 individual dishes. Chill until set. Makes 4 cups (1 L).

1/2 cup (125 mL): 97 Calories; 2.7 g Total Fat (2.5 g Sat., 0.6 mg Cholesterol); 30 mg Sodium; 3 g Protein; 15 g Carbohydrate; trace Dietary Fiber

CHOICES: 1/2 Fruits; 1/2 Other Choices; 1/2 Fats

LEMON FRUIT PUDDING: Layer filling and fresh fruit in individual clear wine glasses or fruit nappies. Chill until set.

LEMON PIE: Pour filling into prepared Graham Bran Pie Crust, page 64. Chill until set.

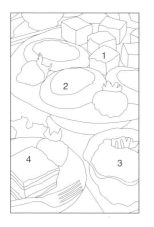

1. Brownies, page 59
2. Mocha Nut Meringues, page 58
3. Blueberry Layered Pudding, page 57
4. Chocolate Éclair Dessert, page 56

Chocolate Éclair Dessert

Amazing how the layers soften overnight into
a cake-like texture. Great creamy chocolate flavour.

Cocoa	1/3 cup	75 mL
Cornstarch	2 tbsp.	30 mL
All-purpose flour	2 tbsp.	30 mL
Granulated sugar	1/2 cup	125 mL
Salt	1/8 tsp.	0.5 mL
Ground cinnamon	1/8 tsp.	0.5 mL
Skim milk	1 cup	250 mL
Can of skim evaporated milk	13 1/2 oz.	385 mL
Frozen egg product, thawed (see Note)	1/2 cup	125 mL
Vanilla	1 tsp.	5 mL
Light liquid topping (such as Nutriwhip)	1 cup	250 mL
Cocoa, sifted	1 tbsp.	15 mL
Graham crackers	28	28
Cocoa, sifted, for garnish	1 tsp.	5 mL

Combine first 6 ingredients in medium saucepan. Slowly whisk in both milks until smooth. Heat and stir on medium until boiling and thickened. Remove from heat.

Add two large spoonfuls of hot cocoa mixture to egg product in small bowl. Mix well. Whisk into cocoa mixture until smooth. Heat for 2 minutes. Stir in vanilla. Cover with plastic wrap directly on the surface to prevent skin from forming. Let stand until cooled to room temperature.

Beat liquid topping with second amount of cocoa in medium bowl until stiff.

Arrange 1/2 of graham crackers in single layer in 9 × 9 inch (22 × 22 cm) pan. Cut to fit if necessary. Whisk cocoa mixture until smooth. Spread 1/2 of cocoa mixture on crackers and spread evenly. Spread 1/2 of topping mixture on cocoa mixture. Cover with single layer of remaining crackers, remaining cocoa mixture and topping mixture. Cover with plastic wrap and refrigerate for 24 hours to allow crackers to soften completely.

Just before serving, sift cocoa over top. For a more decorative look, place doily over top of dessert, then sift with cocoa. Carefully lift and remove doily and excess cocoa. Cuts into 16 pieces.

1 piece: 126 Calories; 2.1 g Total Fat (1 g Sat., 1.2 mg Cholesterol); 158 mg Sodium; 5 g Protein; 23 g Carbohydrate; 1 g Dietary Fibre

CHOICES: 1 Grains & Starches; 1/2 Fats

Pictured on page 54 and on back cover.

Note: 4 tbsp. (50 mL) = 1 large egg

Blueberry Layered Pudding

Frozen cheesecake in a bowl.

Envelope of unflavoured gelatin	1/4 oz.	7 g
Cold water	1/4 cup	60 mL
Non-fat spreadable cream cheese	8 oz.	225 g
Non-fat lemon yogurt	26.8 oz.	750 g
Graham cracker crumbs	2/3 cup	150 mL
Can of blueberry pie filling	19 oz.	540 mL
Light frozen whipped topping, thawed, for garnish	1 cup	250 mL
Grated lemon zest, for garnish		
Fresh blueberries, for garnish		

Stir gelatin into cold water in small saucepan. Let stand for 5 minutes. Heat and stir on low until liquid and gelatin is dissolved. Cool to warm room temperature but still liquid.

Beat cream cheese until smooth. Beat in gelatin and yogurt on very low speed until just mixed. Chill for 1 hour.

Place 1/3 of yogurt mixture in shallow 7 cup (1.75 L) freezer-safe bowl. Sprinkle with 1/3 cup (75 mL) graham crumbs. Spoon 1/2 of pie filling evenly over crumbs. Repeat layers, ending with final 1/3 of yogurt mixture. Swirl with spatula to create marble effect. Freeze for at least 4 hours until firm.

Garnish with whipped topping, lemon zest and fresh blueberries. Serves 8.

1 serving: 286 Calories; 2.3 g Total Fat (1.5 g Sat., 4.0 mg Cholesterol); 270 mg Sodium; 10 g Protein; 57 g Carbohydrate; 2 g Dietary Fibre

CHOICES: 1/2 Grains & Starches; 1 1/2 Other Choices; 1/2 Milk & Alternatives

Pictured on page 54.

Mocha Nut Meringues

Individual desserts for 10 special guests.

Cocoa	2 tsp.	10 mL
Icing (confectioner's) sugar	3 tbsp.	50 mL
Instant coffee granules, ground to fine powder (see Note)	1 1/2 tsp.	7 mL
Vanilla Yogurt Cheese, page 75	2 1/4 cups	550 mL
Egg whites (large), room temperature	3	3
Cream of tartar	1/4 tsp.	1 mL
Salt	1/8 tsp.	0.5 mL
Granulated sugar	1/3 cup	75 mL
Icing (confectioner's) sugar	1/2 cup	125 mL
Ground cinnamon	1/8 tsp.	0.5 mL
Semisweet chocolate baking square, finely grated	1 oz.	28 g
Finely crushed almonds, toasted (see Tip, page 111)	2 tbsp.	30 mL

Combine first 3 ingredients and press through fine meshed sieve into medium bowl. Stir in Vanilla Yogurt Cheese. Cover. Chill. Makes 2 1/4 cups (550 mL).

Beat next 3 ingredients in medium bowl until foamy. Slowly add granulated sugar until soft peaks form. Slowly add icing sugar, 1 tbsp. (15 mL) at a time, until glossy and stiff. Fold in remaining 3 ingredients. Cut parchment paper to fit baking sheets. Draw ten 4 inch (10 cm) ovals on one side. Turn paper over and tape to baking sheets. Pipe egg white mixture onto oval using medium tip. Make thin base, slightly building up sides. Bake in 275°F (140°C) oven for 2 1/2 hours, switching baking sheet positions at half-time. Leave in oven overnight, with door closed, to dry completely and cool. Fill centers of meringues with scant 1/4 cup (60 mL) yogurt mixture just before serving. Makes 10 meringues.

1 meringue: 151 Calories; 3.2 g Total Fat (1.7 g Sat., 6.2 mg Cholesterol); 133 mg Sodium; 7 g Protein; 25 g Carbohydrate; 1 g Dietary Fibre

CHOICES: 1 Other Choices; 1/2 Milk & Alternatives; 1 Fats

Pictured on page 54.

Note: To grind instant coffee granules to a fine powder, crush with back of spoon in a small bowl.

Brownies

These are a very good substitute for high-fat brownies.
They are moist and rich. High in sugar so cut them small,
and only indulge when you must have a sweet chocolate treat.

Frozen egg product, thawed (see Note)	1/2 cup	125 mL
Canola oil	1/4 cup	60 mL
Jar of strained prunes (baby food)	4 1/2 oz.	128 mL
Vanilla	2 tsp.	10 mL
Brown sugar, packed	1/2 cup	125 mL
Granulated sugar	1/2 cup	125 mL
Cocoa	1/2 cup	125 mL
All-purpose flour	2/3 cup	150 mL
Baking powder	1/2 tsp.	2 mL
Salt	1/8 tsp.	0.5 mL
GLAZE (optional)		
Cocoa	1 tbsp.	15 mL
Icing (confectioner's) sugar	1/2 cup	125 mL
Hot water	1 tbsp.	15 mL

Beat first 4 ingredients in large bowl until smooth. Beat in next 3 ingredients. Beat in next 3 ingredients until smooth. Pour next 3 ingredients into greased 8 × 8 inch (20 × 20 cm) baking pan. Bake in 325°F (160°C) oven for 30 to 35 minutes just until center is set. Do not overcook (see Note).

Glaze: Combine all 3 ingredients in small bowl until smooth. Drizzle over warm brownies. Cool. Cuts into 25 squares.

1 square: 78 Calories; 2.6 g Total Fat (0.3 g Sat., 0 mg Cholesterol); 26 mg Sodium; 1 g Protein; 14 g Carbohydrate; 1 g Dietary Fibre

CHOICES: 1/2 Other Choices; 1/2 Fats

Pictured on page 54.

Note: 4 tbsp. (50 mL) = 1 large egg

Note: To prevent overbaking brownies, watch the edges for signs of pulling away from the pan. At that point, if a wooden pick inserted in the center comes out clean but moist, it is done.

Tangy Lemon Spread

Delicious on muffins and as the base for Rainbow Fruit Pizza, page 49.
Try the variation — it makes a great fresh fruit dip.

Cornstarch	2 tbsp.	30 mL
Granulated sugar	1/4 cup	60 mL
Water	1/2 cup	125 mL
Lemon juice (fresh is best)	3 tbsp.	50 mL
Grated lemon zest (optional)	1/4 tsp.	1 mL
Drops of yellow food coloring (optional)	2	2
Non-fat plain yogurt	1 cup	250 mL

Combine cornstarch and sugar in small saucepan. Add water. Heat and stir on medium until boiling and thickened.

Stir in next 3 ingredients. Let cool.

Stir in yogurt. Chill. Makes 1 2/3 cups (400 mL).

1 tbsp. (15 mL): 15 Calories; trace Total Fat (trace Sat., 0.2 mg Cholesterol); 7 mg Sodium; trace Protein; 3 g Carbohydrate; trace Dietary Fibre

CHOICES: None

TANGY LEMON DIP: Fold in 1 cup (250 mL) light frozen whipped topping, thawed, for a fluffy, fresh fruit dip.

Apricot Almond Pudding

A nice change from regular rice pudding. Serve warm or cold.

2% evaporated milk	1 cup	250 mL
Skim milk	2 cups	500 mL
Pearl (or arborio) rice	1/2 cup	125 mL
Salt	1/4 tsp.	1 mL
Ground cinnamon	1/4 tsp.	1 mL
Finely chopped dried apricots	1/3 cup	75 mL
Grated lemon zest (optional)	1 tsp.	5 mL
Sugar substitute (such as Sugar Twin)	1 tbsp.	15 mL
Almond flavouring	1/4 tsp.	1 mL
Toasted crushed almonds (optional), see Tip, page 111	1 tbsp.	15 mL

(continued on next page)

Desserts

Combine first 6 ingredients in top of double boiler. Heat over boiling water for about 45 minutes, stirring occasionally, until thickened and creamy.

Stir in next 3 ingredients. Sprinkle with almonds. Makes 3 cups (750 mL).

1/2 cup (125 mL): 152 Calories; 1.2 g Total Fat (0.7 g Sat., 5.0 mg Cholesterol); 208 mg Sodium; 8 g Protein; 28 g Carbohydrate; 1 g Dietary Fibre

CHOICES: 1 Grains & Starches; 1/2 Milk & Alternatives

RAISIN PUDDING: Omit apricots and almond flavouring. Add 1/3 cup (75 mL) raisins and 1/4 tsp. (1 mL) vanilla. Sprinkle with cinnamon.

Sour Fruit Pops

Tart flavour will remind you of sour candies! A refreshing
frozen treat for hot summer days or birthday parties.

Chopped fresh rhubarb	1 1/2 cups	375 mL
Water	2/3 cup	150 mL
Package of regular (or sugar-free)	3 oz.	85 g
strawberry-flavoured gelatin (jelly powder)		
Chopped fresh strawberries	1 1/2 cups	375 mL
Non-fat vanilla yogurt	1/2 cup	125 mL

Cook rhubarb in water in small saucepan for 10 minutes, stirring frequently, until softened. Stir in jelly powder until dissolved. Pour into blender.

Add strawberries and yogurt. Process until smooth. Pour 1/4 cup (60 mL) into each freezer pop form and insert handles. Freeze until solid. Makes 12 fruit pops.

1 fruit pop: 41 Calories; 0.1 g Total Fat (trace Sat., 0.2 mg Cholesterol); 29 mg Sodium; 1 g Protein; 9 g Carbohydrate; 1 g Dietary Fibre

CHOICES: 1/2 Other Choices

Variation: Pour 1/2 cup (125 mL) of mixture into 6 small waxed paper cups. Insert wooden stick when partially frozen.

Paré Pointer

The boss at the dairy would be the big cheese.

Pumpkin Mousse In A Ginger Crust

Makes two pies for company. Delicious served frozen.

Gingersnap crumbs (see Note)	3 cups	750 mL
Margarine, melted	1/2 cup	125 mL
Brown sugar, packed	1/3 cup	75 mL
Salt	1/4 tsp.	1 mL
Ground nutmeg	1/4 tsp.	1 mL
Ground ginger	1/2 tsp.	2 mL
Ground cinnamon	1/2 tsp.	2 mL
Envelopes of unflavoured gelatin (1/4 oz., 7 g, each)	2	2
Skim evaporated milk	3/4 cup	175 mL
Frozen egg product, thawed (see Note)	1/2 cup	125 mL
Can of pumpkin (without spices)	14 oz.	398 mL
Egg whites (large), room temperature	3	3
Granulated sugar	1/4 cup	60 mL

Combine gingersnap crumbs and margarine in medium bowl. Pack into bottom and up sides of two 9 inch (22 cm) pie plates. Bake in 350°F (175°C) oven for 8 to 10 minutes until firm. Cool.

Combine next 6 ingredients in medium saucepan. Slowly stir in next 3 ingredients. Whisk together until smooth. Heat and stir on medium until thickened and gelatin is dissolved. Chill, stirring occasionally, until mixture mounds when dropped from spoon.

Beat egg whites in large clean bowl until soft peaks start to form. While beating, add granulated sugar, 1 tbsp. (15 mL) at a time, until stiff peaks form. Fold in pumpkin mixture. Divide filling between two crusts. Chill for several hours or overnight to set. Each pie cuts into 8 wedges, for a total of 16.

1 wedge: 224 Calories; 8.2 g Total Fat (1.9 g Sat., 8.3 mg Cholesterol); 306 mg Sodium; 5 g Protein; 33 g Carbohydrate; 1 g Dietary Fibre

CHOICES: 1 1/2 Grains & Starches; 1 1/2 Fats

Note: 4 tbsp. (50 mL) = 1 large egg

Note: To make gingersnap crumbs, process whole cookies in food processor or blender until desired consistency.

FROZEN PUMPKIN DESSERT: Reserve 1/2 cup (125 mL) crumbs. Combine remainder with margarine and pack in bottom and up sides of 10 inch (25 cm) springform pan or bottom of 9 x 13 inch (22 x 33 cm) pan. Pour in filling. Sprinkle with reserved crumbs. Chill to set. Freeze.

Peach Packages

A perfect amount of peach filling is encased in layers of pastry.

Chopped fresh (or frozen, thawed) peaches	2 cups	500 mL
Lemon juice	1 tbsp.	15 mL
Brown sugar, packed	1 tbsp.	15 mL
Raisins	2 tbsp.	30 mL
Ground cinnamon	1/2 tsp.	2 mL
Ground ginger	1/4 tsp.	1 mL
Minute tapioca	2 tsp.	10 mL
Fine dry whole wheat bread crumbs (see Tip, page 80)	2 tbsp.	30 mL
Brown sugar, packed	1 1/2 tsp.	7 mL
Ground cinnamon	1/4 tsp.	1 mL
Frozen phyllo pastry sheets, thawed	12	12
No-stick cooking spray		
Granulated sugar (optional)	1 tsp.	5 mL
Ground cinnamon (optional)	1/16 tsp.	0.5 mL

Combine first 7 ingredients in medium bowl. Let stand for 10 minutes.

Mix next 3 ingredients in small bowl.

Lay 1 sheet phyllo on flat surface. Sprinkle with 1/2 tbsp. (7 mL) bread crumb mixture. Cover with second sheet. Fold in half widthwise. Spoon 1/6 of peach mixture (generous 1/3 cup, 75 mL) about 2 inches (5 cm) from narrow end, leaving about 2 inches (5 cm) phyllo on either side. Roll edge over pastry. Tuck in sides and continue rolling until filling is completely enclosed. Place seam side down on lightly sprayed baking sheet. Repeat to make 5 more packages.

Spray packages with no-stick cooking spray. Lightly sprinkle with sugar and cinnamon. Bake in 375°F (190°C) oven for 20 minutes until golden brown. Makes 6 packages.

1 package: 208 Calories; 1.2 g Total Fat (0.2 g Sat., trace Cholesterol); 290 mg Sodium; 5 g Protein; 46 g Carbohydrate; 2 g Dietary Fibre

CHOICES: 2 Grains & Starches; 1/2 Fruits

APPLE CRANBERRY PACKAGES: Omit peaches. Add 2 medium apples, peeled and sliced, and 1/3 cup (75 mL) chopped dried cranberries.

Strawberry Banana Frozen Yogurt

Try customizing the flavour by using different fruit.

Ripe medium banana	1	1
Whole fresh strawberries (5 large or 10 medium)	6 oz.	170 g
Non-fat vanilla yogurt	1 cup	250 mL
Lemon juice	1 tsp.	5 mL
Liquid honey	1 1/2 tsp.	7 mL
Vanilla	1/2 tsp.	2 mL
Light frozen whipped topping, thawed	1 cup	250 mL

Cut banana into 1 inch (2.5 cm) chunks. Arrange with strawberries in single layer on baking sheet. Freeze for about 2 hours until hard.

Process frozen fruit with next 4 ingredients in food processor until slushy and smooth.

Fold in whipped topping. Empty into freezer container. Freeze for at least 3 hours. Stir well every 1/2 hour for the first 1 1/2 hours. Makes 3 1/2 cups (875 mL).

1/2 cup (125 mL): 73 Calories; 1.7 g Total Fat (1.5 g Sat., 0.7 mg Cholesterol); 30 mg Sodium; 2 g Protein; 13 g Carbohydrate; 1 g Dietary Fibre

CHOICES: 1/2 Fruits

Graham Bran Pie Crust

Crisp, nutty flavour. Use Lemon Chiffon Filling, page 55, for a light, fluffy pie.

Graham cracker crumbs	1 1/4 cups	300 mL
All-bran cereal	1/2 cup	125 mL
Margarine, melted	1 tbsp.	15 mL
Non-fat vanilla yogurt	2 tbsp.	30 mL
Orange juice	1 tbsp.	15 mL
Ground cinnamon	1/4 tsp.	1 mL
Ground nutmeg, sprinkle		

Blend or process graham crumbs and cereal until very finely ground. Empty into medium bowl.

(continued on next page)

Stir in remaining 5 ingredients. Press into greased 9 inch (22 cm) pie plate. Bake in center of 325°F (160°C) oven for 8 to 10 minutes until set. Remove before too brown. Makes one 9 inch (22 cm) pie crust.

1/8 crust: 95 Calories; 3.1 g Total Fat (0.7 g Sat., 0.1 mg Cholesterol); 179 mg Sodium; 2 g Protein; 17 g Carbohydrate; 2 g Dietary Fibre

CHOICES: 1 Grains & Starches; 1/2 Fats

Creamy Rice Pudding

Very creamy with minimal fat from the 2% milk.
Using skim milk will produce a curdled pudding.

Can of skim evaporated milk	13 1/2 oz.	385 mL
2% milk	2 cups	500 mL
Cooked white rice	2 cups	500 mL
Liquid honey	1/4 cup	60 mL
Ground cinnamon	1/4 tsp.	1 mL
Salt	1/4 tsp.	1 mL
Light (or sultana) raisins	1/3 cup	75 mL
Frozen egg product, thawed (see Note)	1/2 cup	125 mL
Vanilla	2 tsp.	10 mL

Combine first 7 ingredients in large uncovered saucepan. Bring to a boil. Reduce heat. Simmer, uncovered, for 15 minutes, stirring frequently.

Measure egg product into small bowl. Add 1/2 cup (125 mL) hot mixture to egg. Mix well. Stir into saucepan. Heat, stirring constantly, until thickened.

Remove from heat. Stir in vanilla. Cover with plastic wrap directly on surface to prevent skin from forming. Serve warm or cooled to room temperature. Makes 5 1/4 cups (1.3 L).

1/2 cup (125 mL): 158 Calories; 1.2 g Total Fat (0.7 g Sat., 5.1 mg Cholesterol); 160 mg Sodium; 7 g Protein; 30 g Carbohydrate; 1 g Dietary Fibre

CHOICES: 1 Grains & Starches

Note: 4 tbsp. (50 mL) = 1 large egg

Ginger Lime Dip

A delightfully fresh taste to dip fresh fruit in.

Yogurt Cheese, page 75	1/2 cup	125 mL
Liquid honey	1 tbsp.	15 mL
Lime juice	1 tbsp.	15 mL
Grated lime zest	1/4 tsp.	1 mL
Light frozen whipped topping, thawed	1/2 cup	125 mL
Ground ginger	1/4 tsp.	1 mL

Combine all 6 ingredients in small dish. Whisk until blended. Makes 3/4 cup (175 mL).

1 tbsp. (15 mL): 26 Calories; 0.8 g Total Fat (0.6 g Sat., 1.2 mg Cholesterol); 15 mg Sodium; 1 g Protein; 4 g Carbohydrate; trace Dietary Fibre

CHOICES: None

Milk Chocolate Sauce

Great served on a scoop of vanilla frozen yogurt.

Cocoa	2 tbsp.	30 mL
Vanilla custard powder	2 tbsp.	30 mL
Granulated sugar	2 tbsp.	30 mL
Can of skim evaporated milk	13 1/2 oz.	385 mL
Margarine	1 tbsp.	15 mL
Vanilla	2 tsp.	10 mL

Combine first 3 ingredients in small saucepan. Slowly whisk in evaporated milk until smooth. Add margarine. Heat and stir on medium until boiling and slightly thickened (see Note). Remove from heat.

Stir in vanilla. Makes 1 1/2 cups (375 mL).

2 tbsp. (30 mL): 55 Calories; 1.1 g Total Fat (0.3 g Sat., 1.2 mg Cholesterol); 57 mg Sodium; 3 g Protein; 9 g Carbohydrate; trace Dietary Fibre

CHOICES: None

Note: To prevent milk from scorching, cook sauce in top pan of double boiler over boiling water. Or heat mixture in microwave on medium-high (80%), stirring frequently, until boiling and slightly thickened.

Fruit Crumble

Good fruity flavour with a crunchy topping. Serve with vanilla frozen yogurt.

Can of sliced peaches in pear juice, with juice	14 oz.	398 mL
Pitted prunes (about 2/3 cup, 150 mL)	15	15
Whole wheat flour	1/3 cup	75 mL
Quick-cooking rolled oats (not instant)	1/3 cup	75 mL
Brown sugar, packed	2 tbsp.	30 mL
Salt	1/4 tsp.	1 mL
Margarine	2 tbsp.	30 mL

Pour peaches with juice into lightly greased 1 quart (1 L) shallow baking dish or 8 x 8 inch (20 x 20 cm) pan. Arrange prunes on peaches.

Combine next 4 ingredients in medium bowl. Cut in margarine until mixture is crumbly. Sprinkle evenly over fruit. Bake, uncovered, in 350°F (175°C) oven for 35 to 40 minutes until browned. Makes 2 3/4 cups (675 mL).

1/2 cup (125 mL): 194 Calories; 4.9 g Total Fat (1.0 g Sat., 0 mg Cholesterol); 183 mg Sodium; 3 g Protein; 38 g Carbohydrate; 4 g Dietary Fibre

CHOICES: 1 Grains & Starches; 1 Fruits; 1 Fats

Fresh Fruit Salad

Serve by itself or over Lemon Cheesecake, page 48. Has a lovely sauce that forms while marinating in the refrigerator.

Sliced fresh strawberries	1 cup	250 mL
Diced cantaloupe	1 cup	250 mL
Medium oranges, peeled, halved and thinly sliced	2	2
Kiwifruit, peeled and diced	2	2
Sugar-free lemon-lime soft drink	3/4 cup	175 mL
Medium banana, diced	1	1

Combine first 4 ingredients in medium bowl. Pour soft drink over top. Toss lightly. Cover. Chill for 1 hour to blend flavours.

Mix in banana. Makes 3 cups (750 mL).

1/2 cup (125 mL): 66 Calories; 0.4 g Total Fat (trace Sat., 0 mg Cholesterol); 6 mg Sodium; 1 g Protein; 16 g Carbohydrate; 3 g Dietary Fibre

CHOICES: 1 Fruits

Lemon Angel Tower

This makes an elegant birthday cake.
A serrated knife works best to cut angel food cake.

Package of angel food cake mix	16 oz.	450 g
FROSTING		
Package of lemon-flavoured gelatin (jelly powder), see Note	3 oz.	85 g
Boiling water	1/2 cup	125 mL
Non-fat lemon yogurt	3/4 cup	175 mL
Light liquid topping (such as Nutriwhip)	1 cup	250 mL
Grated zest from 1 medium lemon		
Strips of lemon zest, for garnish		

Prepare angel food cake as per package directions. Cool completely. Slice horizontally twice to make 3 equal layers.

Frosting: Dissolve jelly powder in boiling water in small bowl. Whisk in yogurt until smooth. Chill about 30 minutes, stirring every 10 minutes, until syrupy.

Beat liquid topping until stiff peaks form. Add lemon zest. Gradually add yogurt mixture while beating. Chill for about 40 minutes, folding several times, until set to spreadable consistency. Makes 6 cups (1.5 L) frosting.

Fill each layer with about 1 1/2 cups (375 mL) frosting. Use remaining frosting to cover top and sides of cake. Garnish with lemon zest. Chill. Cuts into 20 wedges.

1 wedge: 117 Calories; 0.6 g Total Fat (0.5 g Sat., 0.2 mg Cholesterol); 63 mg Sodium; 3 g Protein; 26 g Carbohydrate; trace Dietary Fibre

CHOICES: 1 Grains & Starches; 1/2 Other Choices

Note: To further reduce sugar, use sugar-free lemon-flavoured gelatin (jelly powder).

Paré Pointer

Bananas use suntan lotion because they peel.

Parkerhouse Pockets

Golden, cheese-filled rolls delicious with salad or as part of a brunch.

Light ricotta cheese	8 oz.	250 g
Green onions, finely sliced	4	4
Small potato, peeled, cooked and mashed	1	1
Skim milk	1 1/4 cups	300 mL
Granulated sugar	1/3 cup	75 mL
Canola oil	1/4 cup	60 mL
Salt	3/4 tsp.	4 mL
Whole wheat flour	2 cups	500 mL
Package of instant yeast (or 2 1/4 tsp., 11 mL, bulk)	1/4 oz.	8 g
Egg white (large), fork-beaten	1	1
All-purpose flour	2 – 2 1/2 cups	500 – 625 mL

Combine ricotta and green onion in small bowl. Set aside.

Combine next 5 ingredients in small saucepan. Heat and stir on medium until sugar is dissolved. Cool until very warm but not hot.

Combine whole wheat flour and yeast in large bowl. Stir in potato mixture until thick batter consistency. Add egg white. Mix well. Add all-purpose flour, 1/2 cup (125 mL) at a time, until soft dough is formed. Turn out and knead on floured surface for about 10 minutes until smooth and elastic. Cover. Let rest 15 minutes in oven with light on and door closed. Cut dough in half. Roll one portion out on lightly floured surface to scant 1/2 inch (12 mm) thickness. Cut with 3 inch (7 cm) round cutter. Fill middle with 1 tsp. (5 mL) cheese mixture. Fold over and pinch side like perogy. Repeat with remaining dough. Arrange pockets on 2 large greased baking sheets. Cover. Let rise in oven with light on and door closed for 40 minutes until doubled in size. Bake in 350°F (175°C) oven for 20 to 25 minutes until golden brown. Makes 24 pockets.

1 pocket: 144 Calories; 3.6 g Total Fat (0.8 g Sat., 3.5 mg Cholesterol); 108 mg Sodium; 5 g Protein; 24 g Carbohydrate; 2 g Dietary Fibre

CHOICES: 1 Grains & Starches; 1/2 Fats

Pictured on page 71.

Tuna Toast

Deliciously different for lunch or brunch.

Whole wheat bread slices	4	4
Margarine (optional)	4 tsp.	20 mL
Can of white tuna, packed in water, drained and flaked	6 oz.	170 g
Fresh asparagus, cooked (or 1 can, 12 oz., 341 mL, drained)	8 oz.	225 g
Egg whites (large)	2	2
Light salad dressing (or low-fat mayonnaise)	1/4 cup	60 mL
Chili sauce	1 tbsp.	15 mL
Paprika, sprinkle		

Toast bread slices. Spread one side of each with 1 tsp. (5 mL) margarine if desired.

Spread 1/4 of tuna on buttered side of each slice of toast. Top with asparagus. Place on baking sheet.

Beat egg whites in medium bowl until very stiff. Fold in salad dressing and chili sauce. Divide and spread egg white mixture right to edges over tuna and asparagus. Sprinkle with paprika. Bake in 400°F (205°C) oven on center rack for 8 minutes until topping is golden. Cut diagonally into 4 pieces.

1 piece: 190 Calories; 5.8 g Total Fat (0.6 g Sat., 17.0 mg Cholesterol); 506 mg Sodium; 16 g Protein; 20 g Carbohydrate; 3 g Dietary Fibre

CHOICES: 1 Grains & Starches; 2 Meat & Alternatives

Variation: Omit asparagus. Cut medium tomato into 1/2 inch (12 mm) slices. Arrange on tuna.

Pictured at right.

1. Parkenhouse Pockets, page 69
2. Lemonberry Smoothie, page 25
3. Individual Pizzas, page 74
4. Tuna Toast, above

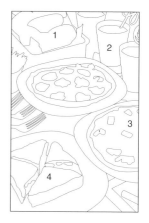

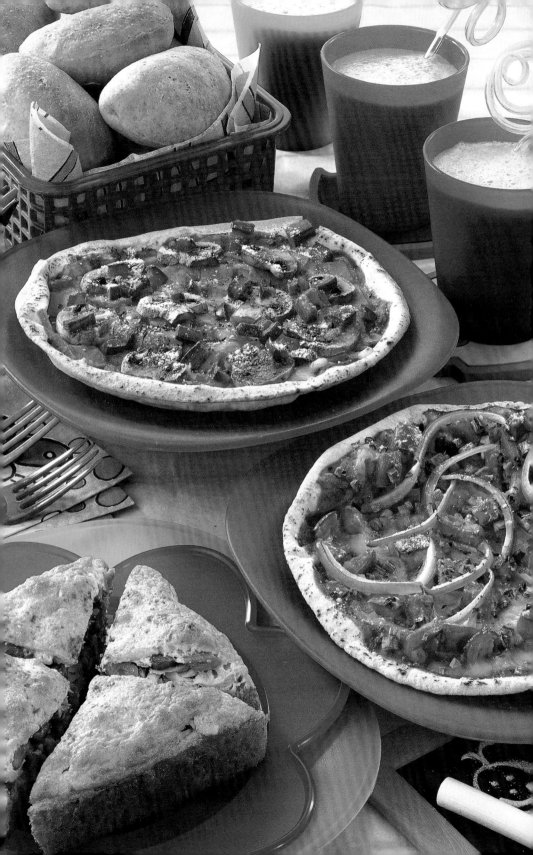

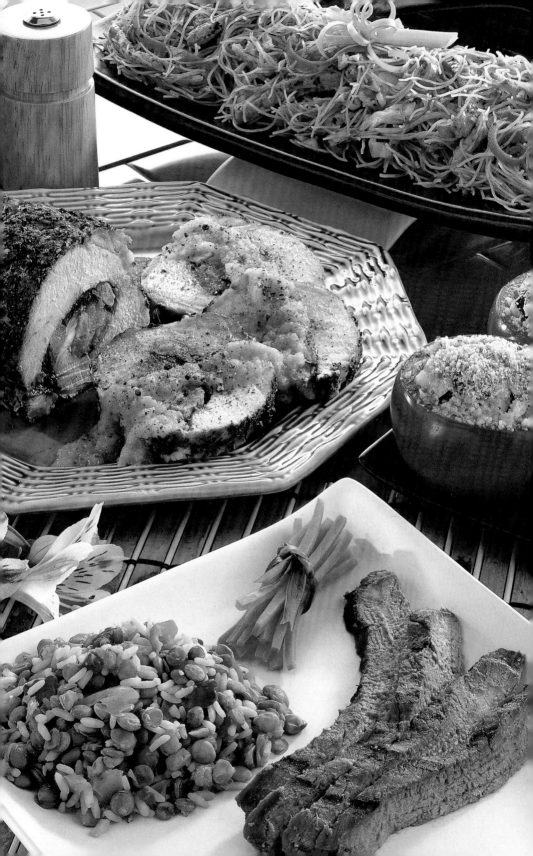

Chicken In Peppers

Can be used as an appetizer or a brunch/lunch offering.

Lean ground chicken	8 oz.	225 g
Thinly sliced green onion	2 tbsp.	30 mL
Finely chopped celery	2 tbsp.	30 mL
Garlic clove, minced	1	1
Cornstarch	2 tsp.	10 mL
Ground ginger	1/2 tsp.	2 mL
Sherry (or alcohol-free sherry)	2 tsp.	10 mL
Black Bean Sauce, page 86 (or commercial)	2 tbsp.	30 mL
Large peppers (your choice of colour, or mixed)	2	2
Toasted sesame seeds (see Tip, page 111)	1 tbsp.	15 mL

Combine first 8 ingredients in small bowl.

Cut peppers in 1/2 crosswise and then quarter each half to make little cups. Remove seeds. Pack about 1 1/2 tsp. (7 mL) chicken mixture in each pepper piece. Place on rack over boiling water or in bamboo steamer. Steam for 8 to 10 minutes until chicken is cooked and peppers are bright green and tender-crisp.

Sprinkle with sesame seeds. Makes 16 pieces.

1 piece: 29 Calories; 0.5 g Total Fat (0.1 g Sat., 8.2 mg Cholesterol); 33 mg Sodium; 4 g Protein; 2 g Carbohydrate; trace Dietary Fibre

CHOICES: 1/2 Meat & Alternatives

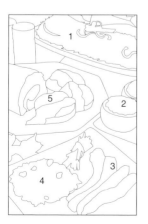

1. Pad Thai, page 94
2. Stuffed Tomatoes, page 134
3. Grilled Hoisin Flank Steak, page 109
4. Lentil Rice, page 139
5. Fruit-Stuffed Pork Loin, page 82

Individual Pizzas

Pizzas that taste great and are quick to make using staples
you have in your home. Don't limit yourself to these toppings.
Try any combination that appeals to you.

Pizza sauce	1 tbsp.	15 mL
Pita bread (7 – 8 inch, 18 – 20 cm, size)	1	1
Grated part-skim mozzarella cheese	1/3 cup	75 mL

VEGETARIAN TOPPING

Garlic powder	1/8 tsp.	0.5 mL
Small Roma (plum) tomato, seeded and diced (about 1/3 cup, 75 mL)	1	1
Finely slivered red onion	2 tbsp.	30 mL
Medium fresh mushrooms, finely diced (about 2 tbsp., 30 mL)	2	2
Dried sweet basil, crushed	1/8 tsp.	0.5 mL
Grated light Parmesan cheese	1 tsp.	5 mL

HAM AND MUSHROOM TOPPING

Fat-free ham slice (3/4 oz., 21 g), diced	1	1
Medium fresh mushrooms (about 1/3 cup, 75 mL), sliced	3	3
Finely diced green pepper	1 tbsp.	15 mL
Grated light Parmesan cheese	1 tsp.	5 mL
Freshly ground pepper, sprinkle		

Spread pizza sauce on pita to edges. Sprinkle cheese evenly over pizza sauce.

Topping (Vegetarian or Ham And Mushroom): Layer toppings over pizza sauce in order given. Place on baking sheet. Bake, uncovered, in 400°F (205°C) oven on center rack for 10 minutes until crispy and browned. Makes 1 pizza.

1 vegetarian pizza: 314 Calories; 8.1 g Total Fat (4.5 g Sat., 24.3 mg Cholesterol); 526 mg Sodium; 18 g Protein; 43 g Carbohydrate; 2 g Dietary Fibre

1 ham and mushroom pizza: 309 Calories; 7.9 g Total Fat (4.5 g Sat., 24.3 mg Cholesterol); 781 mg Sodium; 20 g Protein; 39 g Carbohydrate; 1 g Dietary Fibre

CHOICES: 1 vegetarian pizza: 2 Grains & Starches; 1 1/2 Vegetables; 1 1/2 Meat & Alternatives

CHOICES: 1 ham and mushroom pizza: 2 Grains & Starches; 1/2 Vegetables; 2 Meat & Alternatives

Pictured on page 71.

Spicy Refried Beans

Spread on flour tortillas and heat in the microwave for a delicious bean burrito.

Chopped onion	1/2 cup	125 mL
Garlic clove, minced	1	1
Water	1 tbsp.	15 mL
Brown sugar, packed	1 tsp.	5 mL
Canola oil	1 tsp.	5 mL
Chili powder	1/2 tsp.	2 mL
Cayenne pepper	1/8 tsp.	0.5 mL
Can of pinto beans, with liquid	14 oz.	398 mL
Apple cider vinegar	2 tsp.	10 mL
Salt	1/8 tsp.	0.5 mL

Sauté first 4 ingredients in canola oil in non-stick frying pan on medium-low for about 15 minutes until onion is golden and very soft. Stir in chili powder and cayenne. Sauté for 1 to 2 minutes.

Drain beans, reserving 1/4 cup (60 mL) liquid. Process remaining 3 ingredients in food processor or blender until mushy. Add to onion mixture. Heat on medium-low for 2 to 3 minutes until mixture is dry and paste-like. Makes 1 1/3 cups (325 mL).

1/4 cup (60 mL): 79 Calories; 1.2 g Total Fat (0.1 g Sat., 0 mg Cholesterol); 388 mg Sodium; 4 g Protein; 14 g Carbohydrate; trace Dietary Fibre

CHOICES: 1 Grains & Starches; 1/2 Meat & Alternatives

Yogurt Cheese

This thick yogurt is great for spreads, dips and desserts. Use in Tuna Salad Pitas, page 76, or Mocha Nut Meringues, page 58.

Low-fat plain yogurt, without gelatin	3 2/3 cups	900 mL

Line plastic strainer with a double thickness of cheesecloth. Place over deep bowl. Spoon in yogurt. Cover loosely with plastic wrap. Let stand in refrigerator for 24 hours, discarding liquid in bowl several times. Remove to sealable container. Cover. Store in refrigerator until expiry date on yogurt container. Makes 2 cups (500 mL).

1/4 cup (60 mL): 71 Calories; 1.8 g Total Fat (1.1 g Sat., 6.9 mg Cholesterol); 79 mg Sodium; 6 g Protein; 8 g Carbohydrate; 0 g Dietary Fibre

CHOICES: 1/2 Milk & Alternatives

VANILLA YOGURT CHEESE: Omit low-fat plain yogurt. Use 4 cups (1 L) of low-fat vanilla yogurt. Makes 2 1/8 cups (530 mL).

Lunches

Beef Coleslaw Pitas

Dill pickles give these a bit of tang. Good and crunchy. Fill pita halves just before serving.

Deli roast beef slices, rolled and thinly sliced	6 oz.	170 g
Finely chopped red onion	2 tbsp.	30 mL
Finely diced dill pickle	1/4 cup	60 mL
Finely shredded cabbage	3 cups	750 mL
Grated carrot	1/2 cup	125 mL
DRESSING		
Non-fat plain yogurt	1/4 cup	60 mL
Non-fat salad dressing (or non-fat mayonnaise)	1/4 cup	60 mL
Creamed horseradish	1 tsp.	5 mL
Granulated sugar	1/4 tsp.	1 mL
Salt	1/8 tsp.	0.5 mL
Chopped fresh parsley (optional)	1 tbsp.	15 mL
Pita breads (8 inch, 20 cm, size), cut in half	2	2

Toss first 5 ingredients in medium bowl.

Dressing: Combine first 6 ingredients in small bowl. Toss with cabbage mixture. Makes 4 cups (1 L) filling.

Fill pita halves with 1 cup (250 mL) filling each. Makes 4 pita halves.

1 pita half: 203 Calories; 2.8 g Total Fat (0.9 g Sat., 28.3 mg Cholesterol); 505 mg Sodium; 17 g Protein; 26 g Carbohydrate; 2 g Dietary Fibre

CHOICES: 1 Grains & Starches; 1 Vegetables; 1 1/2 Meat & Alternatives

Tuna Salad Pitas

The Yogurt Cheese offers such a fresh-tasting change from the usual mayonnaise.

Can of white tuna, packed in water, well-drained	4 1/4 oz.	120 g
Diced English cucumber, with peel	1/4 cup	60 mL
Medium Roma (plum) tomato, seeded and diced	1	1
Dill weed	1/4 tsp.	1 mL
Celery salt	1/8 tsp.	0.5 mL
Yogurt Cheese, page 75	1/2 cup	125 mL
Small pita breads (3 inch, 7.5 cm, size)	6	6

Break up tuna with fork in medium bowl. Toss with next 4 ingredients. Stir in Yogurt Cheese.

(continued on next page)

Tear open pitas on one side. Fill with 1/4 cup (60 mL) tuna mixture. Makes 6 pitas.

1 pita: 95 Calories; 1.3 g Total Fat (0.5 g Sat., 10 mg Cholesterol); 179 mg Sodium; 9.0 g Protein; 12 g Carbohydrate; trace Dietary Fibre

CHOICES: 1 Grains & Starches; 1 Meat & Alternatives

Italian Stuffed Peppers

Wild rice and chicken in fleshy, sweet peppers. Yum!

Package of long grain and wild rice mix	6 1/4 oz.	180 g
Chopped onion	1/2 cup	125 mL
Garlic clove, minced	1	1
Chopped fresh mushrooms	1 1/2 cups	375 mL
Grated carrot	1/4 cup	60 mL
Canola oil	1 tsp.	5 mL
Ground chicken breast	10 oz.	280 g
Can of tomato sauce	7 1/2 oz.	213 mL
Chopped fresh sweet basil (or 1 tsp., 5 mL, dried)	2 tbsp.	30 mL
Chopped fresh oregano leaves (or 1/2 tsp., 2 mL, dried)	2 tbsp.	30 mL
Salt	1/4 tsp.	1 mL
Pepper	1/8 tsp.	0.5 mL
Medium green peppers, halved lengthwise	4	4
Water	1/4 cup	60 mL
Grated part-skim mozzarella cheese	1/2 cup	125 mL

Prepare rice as directed on package but without margarine.

Sauté next 4 ingredients in canola oil until soft. Add ground chicken. Scramble-fry until chicken is no longer pink.

Add cooked rice and next 5 ingredients.

Stuff each pepper half with 3/4 cup (175 mL) rice mixture. Place in 9 × 13 inch (22 × 33 cm) pan. Pour water into pan. Cover with foil. Bake in 350°F (175°C) oven for 40 minutes until peppers are tender-crisp.

Remove foil. Top each pepper with 1 tbsp. (15 mL) mozzarella cheese. Bake for 5 minutes until cheese is melted. Makes 8 stuffed peppers.

1 stuffed pepper: 176 Calories; 2.7 g Total Fat (1.0 g Sat., 25.1 mg Cholesterol); 477 mg Sodium; 13 g Protein; 25 g Carbohydrate; 2 g Dietary Fibre

CHOICES: 1 Grains & Starches; 1 Vegetables; 1 Meat & Alternatives

Pizza Pockets

Perfect for eating with your hands. Freeze and reheat for lunches!

Lean ground chicken	8 oz.	225 g
Chopped onion	1 cup	250 mL
Garlic clove, minced	1	1
Grated zucchini, with peel	1 cup	250 mL
Can of regular (or low-sodium) tomato sauce	7 1/2 oz.	213 mL
Dried whole oregano	1/2 tsp.	2 mL
Dried sweet basil	1 tsp.	5 mL
Freshly ground pepper	1/8 tsp.	0.5 mL
Dried crushed chilies	1/8 tsp.	0.5 mL
Grated part-skim mozzarella cheese	3/4 cup	175 mL
Grated light Parmesan cheese	2 tbsp	30 mL
Whole wheat flour	2/3 cup	150 mL
All-purpose flour	1 cup	250 mL
Baking powder	4 tsp.	20 mL
Salt	1/2 tsp.	2 mL
Canola oil	3 tbsp.	50 mL
Skim milk	3/4 cup	175 mL
All-purpose flour	1/3 cup	75 mL
Skim milk	1/4 cup	60 mL

Sauté first 4 ingredients in large non-stick frying pan until no pink remains in ground chicken and liquid is evaporated.

Stir in next 5 ingredients. Heat, uncovered, for 10 minutes on low, stirring occasionally, until thickened. Remove from heat. Let stand to cool slightly. Stir in both cheeses.

Combine next 4 ingredients in medium bowl. Make a well in center.

Combine canola oil and first amount of milk in small bowl. Add, all at once, to dry ingredients. Stir with fork just until moistened.

Turn out and gently knead dough on floured surface, using second amount of all-purpose flour, about 8 to 10 times. Divide dough into 8 portions. Roll each out to 6 inch (15 cm) circle. Place 1/3 cup (75 mL) filling to one side of center. Moisten edge of dough with some of second amount of milk. Bring unfilled side of dough over filling and press edges together with fork tines to seal well. Cut 3 or 4 slits in top with tip of sharp knife. Place on greased baking sheet. Brush with remaining milk. Bake in 400°F (205°C) oven for 13 to 15 minutes until golden brown. Makes 8 pockets.

1 pocket: 263 Calories; 8.2 g Total Fat (1.9 g Sat., 24.2 mg Cholesterol); 464 mg Sodium; 16 g Protein; 32 g Carbohydrate; 3 g Dietary Fibre

CHOICES: 1 1/2 Grains & Starches; 1/2 Vegetables; 1 1/2 Meat & Alternatives; 1 Fats

Pineapple Pork

This flavourful, mildly sweet pork is delicious over brown rice.

Lean boneless pork loin, trimmed and thinly sliced	3/4 lb.	340 g
Canola oil	2 tsp.	10 mL
Paprika	1/2 tsp.	2 mL
Ground ginger	1/2 tsp.	2 mL
Freshly ground pepper, sprinkle		
Medium carrots, thinly sliced on diagonal	2	2
Medium green pepper, cut into large slivers	1/2	1/2
Medium red pepper, cut into large slivers	1/2	1/2
Small onion, sliced lengthwise into wedges	1	1
Can of pineapple tidbits, drained, juice reserved	14 oz.	398 mL
White vinegar	2 tbsp.	30 mL
Brown sugar, packed	1 tbsp.	15 mL
Reserved pineapple juice	1/4 cup	60 mL
Low-sodium soy sauce	1 tbsp.	15 mL
Ketchup	1 tbsp.	15 mL
Cornstarch	2 tbsp.	30 mL

Sauté pork in canola oil in large frying pan for 1 minute. Sprinkle with paprika, ginger and pepper. Sauté until no pink remains in pork.

Stir in next 4 ingredients.

Reserve 1/4 cup (60 mL) pineapple juice. Set aside. Add remaining juice and pineapple to pork mixture. Drizzle with vinegar. Sprinkle with brown sugar. Stir. Bring to a boil. Cover. Simmer for 30 minutes until carrot is tender.

Combine remaining 4 ingredients in small bowl until smooth. Stir into pork mixture. Heat and stir until boiling and thickened. Makes 5 1/4 cups (1.3 L). Serves 4.

1 serving: 274 Calories; 7.5 g Total Fat (1.9 g Sat., 49.7 mg Cholesterol); 279 mg Sodium; 20 g Protein; 32 g Carbohydrate; 3 g Dietary Fibre

CHOICES: 1 Fruits; 1 Vegetables; 3 Meat & Alternatives

Paré Pointer
When the gangsters went sky diving, they had a chute out.

Turkey Vegetable Meatloaf

Have you ever seen a pretty meatloaf? Now you have! Excellent cold in a sandwich.

Medium carrot, cut into chunks	1	1
Medium red pepper, cut into chunks	1	1
Green onions, halved	2	2
Celery rib, cut into chunks	1	1
Garlic clove (optional)	1	1
Skim evaporated milk	1/2 cup	125 mL
Egg whites (large)	3	3
Fine dry whole wheat (or white) bread crumbs (see Tip, below)	1 1/2 cups	375 mL
Seasoned salt	1 tsp.	5 mL
Pepper	1/4 tsp.	1 mL
Worcestershire sauce	1 tsp.	5 mL
Lean ground turkey breast	1 1/4 lbs.	560 g
Can of stewed tomatoes, with juice	14 oz.	398 mL
Chopped fresh parslcy, for garnish		
Red pepper slices, for garnish		

Process first 7 ingredients in food processor or blender until finely chopped. Pour into large bowl.

Add next 5 ingredients. Mix very well. Form into two 8 × 5 inch (20 × 12.5 cm) loaves. Place crosswise in greased or foil-lined 9 × 13 inch (22 × 33 cm) pan.

Process tomatoes with juice until almost puréed. Pour over meatloaves. Bake, uncovered, in 325°F (160°C) oven for 1 1/2 hours. Makes 2 loaves.

Garnish with parsley and red pepper. Serves 8.

1 serving: 204 Calories; 1.6 g Total Fat (0.4 g Sat., 44.2 mg Cholesterol); 554 mg Sodium; 23 g Protein; 23 g Carbohydrate; 1 g Dietary Fibre

CHOICES: 1 Grains & Starches; 2 Vegetables; 3 Meat & Alternatives

Pictured on page 89.

tip — To make 1/4 cup (60 mL) dry whole wheat bread crumbs, remove the crusts from 1 slice of stale or 2-day-old whole wheat bread. Leave the bread on the counter for a day or 2 until it's dry, or, if you're in a hurry, set the bread on a baking sheet and bake in a 200°F (95°C) oven, turning occasionally, until dry. Break the bread into pieces and process until crumbs reach the desired fineness.

Curried Chicken And Bulgur

A delicious one-dish meal. Even leftovers taste good.

Canola oil	2 tsp.	10 mL
Boneless, skinless chicken breast halves (about 3), cut into bite-size pieces	3/4 lb.	340 g
Medium onion, chopped	1	1
Large celery rib, diced	1	1
Medium carrots, coarsely grated	2	2
Curry powder	1/2 tsp.	2 mL
Ground cumin	1/4 tsp.	1 mL
Ground cardamom	1/4 tsp.	1 mL
Can of condensed chicken broth	10 oz.	284 mL
Water	3/4 cup	175 mL
Bulgur wheat (6 oz., 170 g)	1 cup	250 mL
Light raisins	2 tbsp.	30 mL
Ground cinnamon	1/8 tsp.	0.5 mL
Salt	1/8 tsp.	0.5 mL
Finely chopped toasted pecans (see Tip, page 111)	2 tbsp.	30 mL

Heat canola oil in non-stick frying pan on medium-high. Sauté chicken and onion until no pink remains in chicken and onion is soft.

Stir in next 5 ingredients. Heat for about 3 minutes until fragrant and carrot is softened.

Add next 6 ingredients. Cover. Simmer for 15 to 20 minutes until bulgur is tender. Fluff with fork.

Sprinkle with pecans. Makes 5 cups (1.25 L). Serves 4.

1 1/4 cups (300 mL): 334 Calories; 7.4 g Total Fat (1.0 g Sat., 50.1 mg Cholesterol); 646 mg Sodium; 29 g Protein; 40 g Carbohydrate; 9 g Dietary Fibre

CHOICES: 2 Grains & Starches; 1 Vegetables; 3 Meat & Alternatives

Pictured on page 89.

Fruit-Stuffed Pork Loin

Definitely a company dish. The mixed fruit filling complements the pork very well.

Lean boneless pork tenderloin, trimmed (about 8 x 4 x 2 inch, 20 x 10 x 5 cm, size)	2 1/4 lbs.	1 kg
Can of unsweetened applesauce	14 oz.	398 mL
Garlic cloves, minced	3	3
Salt	1/4 tsp.	1 mL
Brown sugar, packed	2 tbsp.	30 mL
Ground cinnamon	1/8 tsp.	0.5 mL
Ground nutmeg	1/16 tsp.	0.5 mL
Boiling water	2 cups	500 mL
Mixed dried fruit (such as apricots, prunes and cranberries), diced	1 cup	250 mL
Canola oil	2 tsp.	10 mL
Dried mixed herbs	1 tbsp.	15 mL
Garlic clove, minced (optional)	1	1
Freshly ground pepper, generous sprinkle		
White wine (or apple juice), optional	1/4 cup	60 mL
SAUCE		
Cornstarch	2 tbsp.	30 mL
Sherry (or non-alcohol sherry)	1/4 cup	60 mL
Ground cinnamon	1/2 tsp.	2 mL
Pepper, sprinkle		

Butterfly tenderloin by cutting horizontally lengthwise, not quite through center. Open flat. Pound with mallet or rolling pin to an even thickness.

Combine 1/3 cup (75 mL) applesauce with garlic and salt in small bowl. Spread on cut side of pork.

Combine next 4 ingredients in medium bowl. Add dried fruit. Let stand for 10 minutes. Drain, reserving liquid. Pack fruit onto pork in even layer, leaving about 1 inch (2.5 cm) from edges on all 4 sides uncovered. Roll jelly roll fashion. Tie with butcher's string or use metal skewers to secure.

Combine next 4 ingredients and 1 tbsp. (15 mL) reserved applesauce mixture in small dish. Coat pork with herb mixture. Place on rack in small roaster or pan with sides. Add wine to bottom of roaster. Cover. Bake in 325°F (160°C) oven for about 1 1/4 hours until internal temperature reaches 160°F (75°C). Remove from oven. Tent with foil.

(continued on next page)

Main Dishes

Sauce: Combine cornstarch and reserved liquid in small saucepan. Add remaining applesauce mixture (about 1 1/4 cups, 300 mL) and sherry. Heat and stir on medium until boiling and thickened. Makes about 2 2/3 cups (650 mL) sauce.

Remove foil from roast. Place on serving platter. Drizzle with sauce. Sprinkle with cinnamon and pepper. Serves 8.

1 serving: 288 Calories; 8.7 g Total Fat (2.7 g Sat., 74.6 mg Cholesterol); 169 mg Sodium; 29 g Protein; 22 g Carbohydrate; 3 g Dietary Fibre

CHOICES: 1 Fruits; 4 Meat & Alternatives

Pictured on page 72.

Barbecued Beef-In-A-Bun

Done in the oven, lean beef is made tender with lots of sauce.

Flank steak, trimmed	1 1/2 lbs.	680 g
Barbecue sauce	1/2 cup	125 mL
Tomato sauce	1/2 cup	125 mL
Garlic cloves, minced (optional)	2	2
Prepared mustard	1 tbsp.	15 mL
Worcestershire sauce	1 tsp.	5 mL
Chopped green pepper	1/2 cup	125 mL
Small onion, thinly sliced	1	1
Whole wheat buns, toasted	8 – 10	8 – 10

Lay steak in bottom of lightly sprayed small roaster or 3 quart (3 L) casserole.

Combine next 6 ingredients in small bowl. Pour over steak.

Top with onion. Cover. Bake in 300°F (150°C) oven for about 2 hours until meat is very tender. Remove steak. Let cool slightly. Thinly slice on diagonal. Return to roaster. Stir.

Pile about 1/3 cup (75 mL) steak and sauce onto each bun to serve. Makes 3 1/2 cups (875 mL).

1/3 cup (75 mL): 191 Calories; 5.9 g Total Fat (2.3 g Sat., 26.4 mg Cholesterol); 393 mg Sodium; 17 g Protein; 17 g Carbohydrate; 3 g Dietary Fibre

CHOICES: 1 Grains & Starches; 2 Meat & Alternatives

To Make Ahead: Fill buns and wrap in plastic wrap and foil. Label. Freeze. To serve, defrost at room temperature for 3 1/2 to 4 hours. Good cold, or wrap in paper towel and microwave on medium (50%) for 30 seconds to 1 minute until hot.

Turkey Breast With Rice Stuffing

So elegant to serve for special guests. Lots of tasty vegetables in the stuffing.

RICE STUFFING		
Long grain brown rice	1/3 cup	75 mL
Wild rice	1/3 cup	75 mL
Boiling water	2 1/3 cups	575 mL
Chicken bouillon powder	1 tbsp.	15 mL
Large onion, chopped	1	1
Chopped fresh mushrooms	2 cups	500 mL
Margarine	2 tbsp.	30 mL
Coarsely grated carrot	1 cup	250 mL
Diced red pepper	2/3 cup	150 mL
Chopped fresh parsley (or 1 tbsp., 15 mL, flakes)	3 tbsp.	50 mL
Finely chopped fresh sweet basil (or 1/2 tsp., 2 mL, dried)	1 tbsp.	15 mL
Grated lemon zest (optional)	1 tsp.	5 mL
Egg white (large)	1	1
Boneless, skinless turkey breast halves (about 2 1/2 lbs., 1.1 kg), see Note	2	2
Water	1/4 cup	60 mL
White (or alcohol-free) wine	1/4 cup	60 mL
Bay leaf	1	1
Freshly ground pepper, sprinkle		
Cornstarch (optional)	1 1/2 tsp.	7 mL

Rice Stuffing: Rinse and drain both rices. Stir into boiling water and bouillon powder in medium saucepan. Cover. Simmer for 40 to 50 minutes until wild rice has popped. Set aside.

Sauté onion and mushrooms in margarine in large frying pan for about 5 minutes until mushrooms have released their juices. Add carrot and red pepper. Sauté for 4 to 5 minutes until vegetables are tender.

Stir in next 3 ingredients. Add rice mixture. Stir in egg white. Makes 4 cups (1 L) stuffing.

Butterfly each turkey breast by cutting horizontally lengthwise, not quite through thickest part. Open flat. Place, 1 at a time, inside heavy plastic bag or between 2 sheets of plastic wrap. Pound with mallet or rolling pin to an even thickness. Remove. Pack 1/2 of stuffing on center of each breast, leaving edges, about 1/2 inch (12 mm), uncovered. Starting with shortest side, roll each breast, enclosing stuffing. Tie at 2 inch (5 cm) intervals with butcher's string. Place seam side down in oval roaster.

(continued on next page)

Pour water and wine on top. Add bay leaf and pepper. Cover. Bake in 350°F (175°C) oven, basting frequently, for 1 1/2 to 1 3/4 hours until internal temperature reaches 175°F (80°C). Let stand in covered roaster for 10 minutes. Remove and discard bay leaf.

Strain juices. Add enough water to equal 2/3 cup (150 mL). Combine with cornstarch in roaster. Heat and stir until boiling and thickened. Makes 2/3 cup (150 mL) sauce. Each roll cuts into 5 slices. Serves 10.

1 serving: 220 Calories; 3.6 g Total Fat (0.8 g Sat., 70.5 mg Cholesterol); 291 mg Sodium; 30 g Protein; 14 g Carbohydrate; 1 g Dietary Fibre

CHOICES: 1 Grains & Starches; 4 Meat & Alternatives

Pictured on page 89.

Note: For 1 large roll (instead of 2 smaller ones), ask the butcher to prepare a whole breast. Flatten as in method. Fill with all the stuffing.

Chicken 'N' Rice

Wholesome flavour in this time-honoured comfort dish. Only 10 minutes to put together, and then forget about it for over an hour!

Boiling water	3 cups	750 mL
Dehydrated mixed vegetables	2/3 cup	150 mL
Chicken bouillon powder	1 tbsp.	15 mL
Garlic clove, minced (optional)	1	1
Poultry seasoning	1/2 tsp.	2 mL
Ground rosemary	1/4 tsp.	1 mL
Celery salt	1/2 tsp.	2 mL
Long grain brown rice	1 1/2 cups	375 mL
Chicken parts, skin removed	1 1/2 lbs.	680 g
Paprika	1/2 tsp.	2 mL
Freshly ground pepper, sprinkle		

Lightly spray 2 quart (2 L) casserole with no-stick cooking spray. Combine first 8 ingredients in casserole.

Arrange chicken over rice mixture. Do not stir. Sprinkle with paprika and pepper. Cover tightly. Bake in 350°F (175°C) oven for 75 minutes. Stir. Cover. Bake for 15 to 20 minutes until rice is tender. Serves 6.

1 serving: 318 Calories; 3.5 g Total Fat (0.8 g Sat., 37.8 mg Cholesterol); 525 mg Sodium; 19 g Protein; 53 g Carbohydrate; 6 g Dietary Fibre

CHOICES: 4 Grains & Starches; 4 Vegetables; 2 1/2 Meat & Alternatives

Chicken And Black Bean Stir-Fry

*Make the sauce a day before so you're all ready to go
for the stir-fry. Serve with brown or white rice.*

BLACK BEAN SAUCE

Dried black beans (see Note)	1/3 cup	75 mL
Boiling water	3 cups	750 mL
Garlic cloves, minced	2	2
Low-sodium soy sauce	1 tbsp.	15 mL
Grated gingerroot	1 tsp.	5 mL
Water	3/4 cup	175 mL
Sherry (or alcohol-free sherry)	2 tbsp.	30 mL
Canola oil	1 tsp.	5 mL
Boneless, skinless chicken breast halves (about 3), cut into long, thin strips	3/4 lb.	340 g
Canola oil	1 tsp.	5 mL
Carrots, thinly cut on diagonal	1/2 cup	125 mL
Broccoli stems, thinly cut on diagonal	2/3 cup	150 mL
Small onion, sliced lengthwise	1	1
Sliced fresh mushrooms	2/3 cup	150 mL
Water	1 tbsp.	15 mL
Broccoli florets, cut into bite-size pieces	1 1/2 cups	375 mL
Fresh pea pods (about 4 oz., 113 g)	20	20

Black Bean Sauce: Cook beans in boiling water in small uncovered saucepan for 70 minutes. Drain. Rinse. Remove 3 tbsp. (50 mL). Freeze remainder in 3 tbsp. (50 mL) portions for future sauce.

Bring beans and next 5 ingredients to a boil in small uncovered saucepan. Boil for about 15 minutes until reduced by half. Mash beans slightly with back of spoon while cooking. Makes 1/3 cup (75 mL) sauce.

Heat first amount of canola oil in non-stick frying pan or wok. Stir-fry chicken on high for 2 to 3 minutes until no pink remains in chicken. Remove to plate.

Heat second amount of canola oil in same frying pan or wok. Stir-fry carrot and broccoli stems for 2 minutes. Add onion and mushrooms. Stir-fry for 2 minutes. Add remaining 3 ingredients. Stir. Cover. Cook for 2 to 3 minutes until broccoli is tender-crisp. Add Black Bean Sauce and chicken. Stir to coat. Makes 4 1/2 cups (1.1 L).

1 cup (250 mL): 173 Calories; 3.4 g Total Fat (0.5 g Sat., 43.8 mg Cholesterol); 134 mg Sodium; 22 g Protein; 14 g Carbohydrate; 3 g Dietary Fibre

CHOICES: 1 1/2 Vegetables; 2 1/2 Meat & Alternatives

(continued on next page)

Pictured on page 89.

Note: To save time, soak beans overnight. Drain. Bring beans and water to a boil in small uncovered saucepan. Cook on medium for about 55 minutes. To save even more time, use 3 tbsp. (50 mL) rinsed and drained canned black beans. Freeze remainder in small batches for future use.

Curried Chicken And Fruit

Fast and delicious. Serve on couscous or rice.

Boneless, skinless chicken breast halves (about 3), cut into bite-size pieces	3/4 lb.	340 g
Chopped onion	1/2 cup	125 mL
Garlic cloves, minced	2	2
Canola oil	2 tsp.	10 mL
Can of stewed tomatoes, with juice, chopped	14 oz.	398 mL
Water	1/2 cup	125 mL
Diced dried apricots	1/4 cup	60 mL
Raisins	1/4 cup	60 mL
Lemon juice	2 tsp.	10 mL
Curry paste (available in Asian section of grocery store)	2 tsp.	10 mL
Chicken bouillon powder	1 tsp.	5 mL
Ground cinnamon	1/4 tsp.	1 mL
Bay leaf	1	1
Skim evaporated milk	1/2 cup	125 mL
Cornstarch	2 tsp.	10 mL

Sauté first 3 ingredients in canola oil in large frying pan for 5 minutes until onion is soft.

Stir in next 9 ingredients. Bring to a boil. Reduce heat. Cover. Simmer for 30 minutes. Remove and discard bay leaf.

Combine evaporated milk and cornstarch in small dish. Add to chicken mixture while stirring. Bring to a boil. Heat for 1 minute until slightly thickened. Makes 4 cups (1 L).

1 cup (250 mL): 244 Calories; 4.4 g Total Fat (0.6 g Sat., 50.6 mg Cholesterol); 533 mg Sodium; 24 g Protein; 28 g Carbohydrate; 3 g Dietary Fibre

CHOICES: 4 Vegetables; 3 Meat & Alternatives

Orange Codfish

This will become your favorite way to do fish! Great with Fresh Fruit Salsa, page 91.

Egg whites (large)	2	2
Frozen concentrated unsweetened orange juice, thawed	3 tbsp.	50 mL
Low-sodium soy sauce	2 tbsp.	30 mL
Fine dry bread crumbs	1/2 cup	125 mL
Parsley flakes	1 tsp.	5 mL
Seasoned salt	1/2 tsp.	2 mL
Lemon pepper	1/2 tsp.	2 mL
Fresh (or frozen, thawed) cod fillets	1 lb.	454 g
Canola oil	1 tbsp.	15 mL
Lemon juice	1 tsp.	5 mL

Beat first 3 ingredients with fork in shallow bowl. Set aside.

Combine next 4 ingredients on sheet of waxed paper.

Dip cod fillets into egg mixture. Coat completely in crumb mixture. Lay in single layer in greased shallow baking dish. Whisk canola oil and lemon juice together in small dish. Drizzle over fish fillets. Bake in 475°F (240°C) oven for 15 to 20 minutes until fish flakes easily. Serves 4.

1 serving: 217 Calories; 4.9 g Total Fat (0.6 g Sat., 49.0 mg Cholesterol); 887 mg Sodium; 25 g Protein; 17 g Carbohydrate; trace Dietary Fibre

CHOICES: 1 Grains & Starches; 3 Meat & Alternatives

Pictured on page 90.

Variation: Omit cod. Use other fish fillets, such as snapper and haddock. Cooking time will be much quicker if very thin fish, such as sole, is used.

1. Chicken And Black Bean Stir-Fry, page 86
2. Turkey Vegetable Meatloaf, page 80
3. Turkey Breast With Rice Stuffing, page 84
4. Curried Chicken And Bulgur, page 81

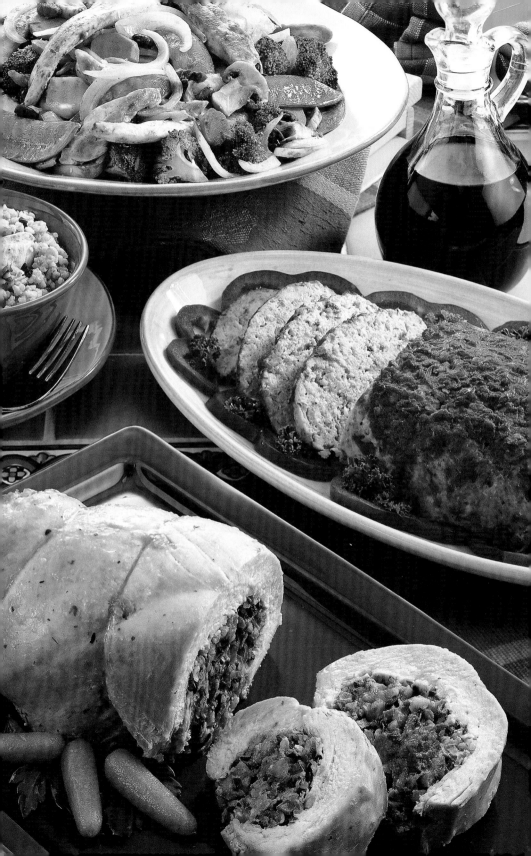

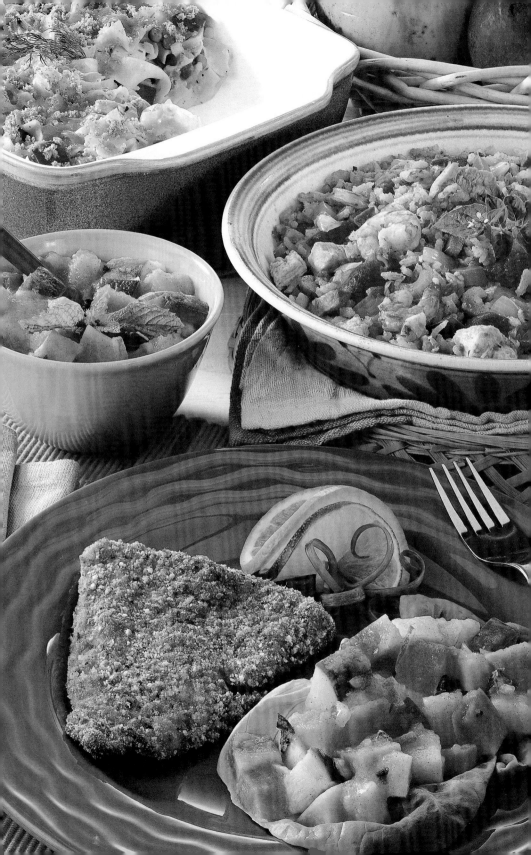

Fresh Fruit Salsa

A very good condiment for roast pork or grilled fish.
Will keep in the refrigerator for up to 4 days.

Medium mango	1	1
Large papaya	1	1
Finely chopped red onion	1/3 cup	75 mL
Small red pepper, diced	1	1
Lime juice	1/3 cup	75 mL
Diced English cucumber, with peel	3/4 cup	175 mL
Chopped fresh cilantro	1 tbsp.	15 mL
Unsweetened applesauce	2/3 cup	150 mL
Granulated sugar	1 tsp.	5 mL
Ground cinnamon	1/4 tsp.	1 mL
Fresh mint, for garnish		

Peel and dice mango and papaya, with juices, into medium bowl.

Stir in next 8 ingredients. Cover. Chill for 1 hour to blend flavours.

Garnish with mint leaves if desired. Makes 3 1/2 cups (875 mL).

1/4 cup (60 mL): 30 Calories; 0.1 g Total Fat (trace Sat., 0 mg Cholesterol); 1 mg Sodium; trace Protein; 8 g Carbohydrate; 1 g Dietary Fibre

CHOICES: 1/2 Fruits

Pictured at left.

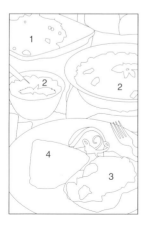

1. Tuna Casserole, page 92
2. Jambalaya, page 93
3. Fresh Fruit Salsa, above
4. Orange Codfish, page 88

Tuna Casserole

An old standby lightened up in calories and fat grams.

Finely chopped onion	2 tbsp.	30 mL
Chopped fresh mushrooms	1/2 cup	125 mL
Diced red pepper	1/2 cup	125 mL
Canola oil	2 tsp.	10 mL
All-purpose flour	2 tbsp.	30 mL
Skim evaporated milk	1 cup	250 mL
Skim milk	1 cup	250 mL
Seasoned salt	1/2 tsp.	2 mL
No-salt herb seasoning	1 tsp.	5 mL
Freshly ground pepper, generous sprinkle		
Frozen peas, thawed and drained	1 cup	250 mL
Can of white tuna, packed in water, drained and broken into chunks	6 oz.	170 g
Medium no-yolk egg noodles	3 cups	750 mL
Water	3 qts.	3 L
Whole wheat bread slice, processed into crumbs	1	1
Grated light sharp Cheddar cheese	1/2 cup	125 mL

Fresh dill, for garnish

Sauté first 3 ingredients in canola oil in large non-stick frying pan until onion is softened. Sprinkle with flour. Stir well. Cook for about 1 minute. Slowly add both milks, stirring constantly, until boiled and just thickened.

Stir in next 3 ingredients. Remove from heat. Stir in peas and tuna.

Cook noodles in boiling water in large uncovered pot or Dutch oven for 8 minutes until tender but firm. Drain well. Pour into greased 2 quart (2 L) casserole. Gently fold in tuna mixture.

Combine bread crumbs and cheese in small bowl. Sprinkle over casserole. Cover. Bake in 350°F (175°C) oven for 30 minutes until bubbling.

Garnish with dill if desired. Serves 6.

1 serving: 248 Calories; 4.9 g Total Fat (1.7 g Sat., 18.5 mg Cholesterol); 400 mg Sodium; 19 g Protein; 32 g Carbohydrate; 2 g Dietary Fibre

CHOICES: 1 Grains & Starches; 1 Vegetables; 1/2 Milk & Alternatives; 1 Meat & Alternatives

Pictured on page 90.

Jambalaya

Add more cayenne pepper or hot pepper sauce for some real Cajun heat!

Olive oil	1 tbsp.	15 mL
Chopped onion	1 cup	250 mL
Chopped celery	1 cup	250 mL
Garlic clove, minced	1	1
Chopped mixed bell peppers	1 cup	250 mL
Boneless, skinless chicken breast halves (about 3), cut into bite-size chunks	3/4 lb.	340 g
Uncooked long grain brown rice	1 1/4 cups	300 mL
Water	2 cups	500 mL
Chicken bouillon powder	1 tbsp.	15 mL
Can of stewed tomatoes, with juice, cut up	14 oz.	398 mL
Hot pepper sauce	1/4 – 1/2 tsp.	1 – 2 mL
Pepper	1/4 tsp.	1 mL
Dried thyme	1/4 tsp.	1 mL
Dried whole oregano	1/4 tsp.	1 mL
Cayenne pepper	1/16 – 1/8 tsp.	0.5 mL
Medium raw shrimp, peeled and deveined (4 oz., 113 g)	12	12
Diced turkey kielbasa (about 3 oz., 85 g)	1/2 cup	125 mL
Sliced green onion	1/4 cup	60 mL

Heat olive oil in large non-stick frying pan. Add next 4 ingredients. Sauté for 5 minutes on medium.

Add chicken and rice. Sauté for 5 minutes until no pink remains in chicken. Turn into lightly sprayed 3 quart (3 L) casserole.

Combine next 8 ingredients in medium saucepan. Bring to a boil. Pour over chicken mixture. Stir gently. Cover. Bake in 350°F (175°C) oven for 45 minutes.

Stir in remaining 3 ingredients. Cover. Bake for 10 minutes until rice is tender. Makes 8 cups (2 L). Serves 6.

1 serving: 331 Calories; 7.5 g Total Fat (1.7 g Sat., 76.9 mg Cholesterol); 797 mg Sodium; 24 g Protein; 42 g Carbohydrate; 4 g Dietary Fibre

CHOICES: 2 Grains & Starches; 2 Vegetables; 2 1/2 Meat & Alternatives; 1/2 Fats

Pictured on page 90.

Pad Thai

*A delicious traditional stir-fry recipe from Thailand. Have the vegetables
cut, noodles softened and sauce made before stir-frying.*

SAUCE		
Fish sauce (available in Asian section of grocery store)	3 tbsp.	50 mL
Water	1/2 cup	125 mL
Chili sauce	1/3 cup	75 mL
Brown sugar, packed	2 tbsp.	30 mL
Low-sodium soy sauce	1/3 cup	75 mL
Cornstarch	4 tsp.	20 mL
Dried crushed chilies (optional)	1/4 tsp.	1 mL
Rice vermicelli, broken	8 oz.	225 g
Cold water, to cover		
Canola oil	2 tsp.	10 mL
Lean boneless pork loin, cut julienne (see Note)	6 oz.	170 g
Garlic cloves, minced	2	2
Shredded cabbage	2 cups	500 mL
Medium carrots, shaved into long, thin ribbons	2	2
Canola oil	1 tsp.	5 mL
Egg whites (large), fork-beaten	2	2
Canola oil	1 tsp.	5 mL
Fresh bean sprouts	1/2 cup	125 mL
Green onions, cut julienne into 4 inch (10 cm) lengths (see Note)	3	3
Chopped fresh parsley (or cilantro)	2 tbsp.	30 mL

Sauce: Combine first 7 ingredients in small bowl. Set aside. Makes about 1 1/2 cups
(375 mL) sauce.

Cover vermicelli with water in large bowl. Let stand for 5 minutes. Drain well.
Set aside.

Heat first amount of canola oil in large non-stick frying pan or wok on medium-high.
Stir-fry pork and garlic for 1 minute. Add cabbage and carrot. Stir-fry for 4 to 5 minutes
until no pink remains in pork and vegetables are tender-crisp. Remove to bowl.

Heat second amount of canola oil in same frying pan. Pour in egg white. Heat,
turning once, until firm. Remove to cutting surface. Slice into long shreds. Add
to pork mixture.

(continued on next page)

Main Dishes

Heat third amount of canola oil in same frying pan. Stir-fry remaining 3 ingredients on medium-high for about 1 minute. Add noodles. Toss. Stir sauce. Add to vegetable mixture. Heat and stir until boiling and slightly thickened. Add pork mixture. Toss until hot. Makes 11 cups (2.75 L). Serves 6.

1 serving: 298 Calories; 4.3 g Total Fat (0.5 g Sat., 16 mg Cholesterol); 1307 mg Sodium; 14 g Protein; 51 g Carbohydrate; 3 g Dietary Fibre

CHOICES: 2 1/2 Grains & Starches; 2 Vegetables; 1 Meat & Alternatives

Pictured on page 72.

Note: It is easier to cut pork into thin strips if slightly frozen.

Asian Chicken Packets

This recipe can easily be doubled or tripled. No dirty pans to wash up after!

Thinly sliced onion	1/2 cup	125 mL
Julienned carrot	3/4 cup	175 mL
Slivered green pepper	1/2 cup	125 mL
Fresh bean sprouts (6 oz., 170 g)	2 cups	500 mL
Couscous	6 tbsp.	100 mL
Boneless, skinless chicken breast halves (about 4 oz., 113 g, each)	2	2
Brown sugar, packed	1 tsp.	5 mL
Ground ginger	1/4 tsp.	1 mL
Garlic powder	1/4 tsp.	1 mL
Hoisin sauce	1 tbsp.	15 mL
Water	3/4 cup	175 mL
Ketchup	1 tbsp.	15 mL
Freshly ground pepper, sprinkle		

Toss first 4 ingredients in medium bowl. Divide between two 12 × 24 inch (30 × 60 cm) heavy-duty foil sheets.

Sprinkle 3 tbsp. (50 mL) couscous on each sheet. Place chicken breast half on top.

Combine next 6 ingredients in small bowl. Drizzle 1/2 (about 7 tbsp., 115 mL, each) on chicken. Sprinkle with pepper. Bring both 12 inch (30 cm) ends up and together over chicken. Fold together several times to seal. Fold sides in at an angle. Roll up to seal and create handles for removing from oven. Repeat for second packet. Cook directly on center rack in 400°F (205°C) oven for 40 minutes. Makes 2 packets.

1 packet: 371 Calories; 2.1 g Total Fat (0.5 g Sat., 65.5 mg Cholesterol); 565 mg Sodium; 35 g Protein; 53 g Carbohydrate; 5 g Dietary Fibre

CHOICES: 2 Grains & Starches; 3 Vegetables; 4 Meat & Alternatives

Indonesian Pork Dinner

Lots of colour and texture to match the variety of flavours in this dish.

Water	3 2/3 cups	900 mL
Vegetable (or chicken) bouillon powder	1 tbsp.	15 mL
Dried crushed chilies	1/4 tsp.	1 mL
Long grain brown rice	1 1/2 cups	375 mL
Chopped onion	1 cup	250 mL
Chopped celery	1 cup	250 mL
Canola oil	2 tsp.	10 mL
Garlic cloves, minced	2	2
Grated gingerroot	2 tsp.	10 mL
Boneless pork loin chops, trimmed and diced	1 lb.	454 g
Ground cumin	1/2 tsp.	2 mL
Curry powder	1 tsp.	5 mL
Diced red pepper	1/4 cup	60 mL
Diced yellow pepper	2/3 cup	150 mL
Frozen mixed vegetables, thawed	3/4 cup	175 mL
Shredded cabbage	2 cups	500 mL
Low-sodium soy sauce	1 1/2 tbsp.	25 mL

Combine first 3 ingredients in large saucepan. Bring to a boil. Stir in rice. Cover. Simmer for 60 to 65 minutes until water is absorbed and rice is tender.

Sauté onion and celery in canola oil in large non-stick frying pan or wok on medium for 2 minutes.

Add next 5 ingredients. Stir-fry for 3 to 4 minutes until no pink remains in pork.

Stir in remaining 5 ingredients. Stir-fry for 3 to 4 minutes until cabbage is softened. Add rice. Toss until rice is steaming hot. Makes 10 cups (2.5 L). Serves 6.

1 serving: 355 Calories; 8 g Total Fat (2.0 g Sat., 44.4 mg Cholesterol); 566 mg Sodium; 23 g Protein; 48 g Carbohydrate; 3 g Dietary Fibre

CHOICES: 2 1/2 Grains & Starches; 1 1/2 Vegetables; 2 Meat & Alternatives

Turkey Cutlets With Mushroom Sauce

Ready in 20 minutes. Serve with rice or noodles.

All-purpose flour	1/4 cup	60 mL
No-salt herb seasoning	1 tbsp.	15 mL
Freshly ground pepper	1/2 tsp.	2 mL
Turkey breast cutlets, cut into 4 portions	1 lb.	454 g
Canola oil	2 tsp.	10 mL
Finely chopped onion	1/4 cup	60 mL
Sliced fresh mushrooms	1 1/2 cups	375 mL
White (or alcohol-free) wine (or chicken broth)	1/2 cup	125 mL
Skim evaporated milk	1/2 cup	125 mL
Cornstarch	2 tsp.	10 mL
Chopped fresh parsley (or 1/2 tsp., 2 mL, flakes)	1 tbsp.	15 mL
Salt	1/4 tsp.	1 mL

Combine first 3 ingredients in small dish. Pour onto waxed paper. Coat both sides of cutlets.

Heat canola oil in large non-stick frying pan on medium-high. Quickly brown both sides of cutlets. Remove to plate.

Sauté onion and mushrooms in same pan on medium, stirring occasionally, until mushroom liquid has evaporated and onion and mushrooms are golden and soft. Add wine. Add cutlets and any accumulated juices from plate. Cover. Simmer for 5 minutes.

Combine remaining 4 ingredients in small dish. Add to pan. Heat and stir for 1 minute until boiling and thickened. Serves 4.

1 serving: 246 Calories; 3.4 g Total Fat (0.5 g Sat., 71.6 mg Cholesterol); 268 mg Sodium; 32 g Protein; 15 g Carbohydrate; 1 g Dietary Fibre

CHOICES: 1/2 Grains & Starches; 4 Meat & Alternatives

Turkey Pot Pie

Great way to use leftover turkey. Double filling
recipe and freeze extra for future use.

FILLING
Water	2 1/2 cups	625 mL
Chicken (or vegetable) bouillon powder	1 tbsp.	15 mL
Diced red potato, with peel	2 cups	500 mL
Chopped celery	1 cup	250 mL
Finely chopped onion	1 cup	250 mL
Dried rosemary, crushed	1/2 tsp.	2 mL
Dried thyme	1/4 tsp.	1 mL
Garlic powder (optional)	1/4 tsp.	1 mL
Freshly ground pepper, sprinkle		
Frozen mixed vegetables	3 cups	750 mL
Chopped, cooked lean turkey (about 3/4 lb., 340 g)	2 cups	500 mL
Skim evaporated milk	2/3 cup	150 mL
All-purpose flour	3 tbsp.	50 mL

CRUST
All-purpose flour	1/2 cup	125 mL
Whole wheat flour	1/2 cup	125 mL
Baking powder	1 1/2 tsp.	7 mL
Salt	1/2 tsp.	2 mL
Canola oil	2 tbsp.	30 mL
Skim milk	1/2 cup	125 mL
Skim milk	1 tbsp.	15 mL
Paprika, sprinkle		

Filling: Combine first 9 ingredients in large uncovered saucepan or Dutch oven. Bring to boil. Cover. Reduce heat. Simmer for 10 minutes.

Add vegetables and turkey. Stir. Cover. Simmer for 15 to 20 minutes until potato is tender.

Whisk evaporated milk into flour in small bowl. Add to turkey mixture. Heat and stir until boiling and thickened. Turn into ungreased 9 × 9 inch (22 × 22 cm) glass pan or 2 1/2 quart (2.5 L) shallow casserole.

Crust: Combine first 4 ingredients in medium bowl.

(continued on next page)

Main Dishes

Add canola oil and skim milk all at once. Stir just until moistened. Turn out onto floured surface. Knead gently 8 to 10 times. Roll out 2/3 of dough to 1/8 inch (3 mm) thickness. Cut into 3/4 to 1 inch (2 to 2.5 cm) wide strips. Lay strips, 1 inch (2.5 cm) apart, diagonally on casserole one way. Roll out scraps and remaining dough. Cut strips as above. Lay on casserole diagonally the other way, creating lattice top.

Brush strips with milk. Sprinkle with paprika. Bake, uncovered, in 400°F (205°C) oven for 15 to 20 minutes until bubbling and top is golden brown. Serves 6.

1 serving: 369 Calories; 7.4 g Total Fat (1.1 g Sat., 57.3 mg Cholesterol); 710 mg Sodium; 28 g Protein; 49 g Carbohydrate; 3 g Dietary Fibre

CHOICES: 2 Grains & Starches; 4 Vegetables; 2 1/2 Meat & Alternatives

Pictured on front cover.

Caesar Chicken

Intense Caesar flavour.

Non-fat mayonnaise (or non-fat salad dressing)	1/4 cup	60 mL
Non-fat Caesar salad dressing	1/4 cup	60 mL
Garlic cloves, minced	2	2
Dry mustard	1/2 tsp.	2 mL
Parsley flakes	1/2 tsp.	2 mL
Freshly ground pepper, sprinkle		
Boneless, skinless chicken breast halves (about 4 oz., 113 g, each)	4	4
Fine dry bread crumbs	1/3 cup	75 mL
Grated light Parmesan cheese	2 tbsp.	30 mL
No-stick cooking spray		

Combine first 6 ingredients in small bowl. Makes 1/2 cup (125 mL) marinade. Transfer to large sealable freezer bag.

Flatten breasts slightly. Place in bag. Turn to coat. Seal. Chill for several hours or overnight.

Combine crumbs and cheese on dinner plate. Remove chicken breasts from bag one at a time, leaving as much dressing mixture on as possible. Coat well in crumb mixture. Place on greased baking sheet. Spray chicken with cooking spray. Bake, uncovered, in center of 375°F (190°C) oven for 25 minutes until no pink remains in chicken and juices run clear. Serves 4.

1 serving: 224 Calories; 4.9 g Total Fat (1.0 g Sat., 69.3 mg Cholesterol); 490 mg Sodium; 29 g Protein; 14 g Carbohydrate; trace Dietary Fibre

CHOICES: 1 Grains & Starches; 4 Meat & Alternatives

Main Dishes

Fast-Fix Beef

Using readily available broccoli slaw makes this very quick.

SAUCE		
Water	1 cup	250 mL
Low-sodium soy sauce	1/4 cup	60 mL
Hoisin sauce	1 tbsp.	15 mL
Cornstarch	2 tbsp.	30 mL
Canola oil	2 tsp.	10 mL
Sirloin steak, trimmed and cut crosswise into very thin slices	3/4 lb.	340 g
Garlic cloves, minced	2	2
Packaged broccoli slaw	3 cups	750 mL
Green onions, sliced	3	3
Fresh (or 10 oz., 285 g, frozen, thawed and drained) pea pods	1 1/4 cups	300 mL
Instant Chinese-style noodles (2 squares), broken up	4 oz.	113 g

Sauce: Combine all 4 ingredients in small bowl. Set aside. Makes about 1 1/2 cups (375 mL) sauce.

Heat canola oil in large frying pan or wok on medium-high. Add beef and garlic. Stir-fry for 1 minute. Add slaw, onion and pea pods. Stir-fry for 3 minutes.

Stir sauce. Add to beef mixture. Stir in noodles. Heat and stir for 3 minutes until boiling and thickened. Makes 6 cups (1.5 L).

1 cup (250 mL): 227 Calories; 6.8 g Total Fat (2.1 g Sat., 41.0 mg Cholesterol); 805 mg Sodium; 19 g Protein; 23 g Carbohydrate; 3 g Dietary Fibre

CHOICES: 1 Grains & Starches; 1 Vegetables; 2 Meat & Alternatives

Mexican Enchiladas

Just a slight bite. Use hot salsa for more spice.

Extra-lean ground beef	1/2 lb.	225 g
Chopped onion	1/2 cup	125 mL
Can of diced green chilies, drained	4 oz.	113 g
Envelope of taco seasoning mix	1/2	1/2
(1 1/4 oz., 35 g)		
Can of pinto beans, drained and rinsed	14 oz.	398 mL
Salsa	1/2 cup	125 mL
Frozen kernel corn	1/3 cup	75 mL
Corn tortillas (6 inch, 15 cm, size)	12	12
Salsa	1/2 cup	125 mL
Grated light sharp Cheddar cheese	1/2 cup	125 mL

Scramble-fry ground beef and onion in large non-stick frying pan until no pink remains in beef.

Stir in next 5 ingredients. Bring to a boil.

Heat tortillas, 6 at a time, wrapped in wet paper towels in microwave on high (100%) for 45 seconds. Place scant 1/3 cup (75 mL) filling on tortilla down center. Fold both sides over filling. Place, folded side down, in lightly greased 9 × 13 inch (22 × 33 cm) pan. Repeat with remaining tortillas. Keep tortillas under damp tea towel or paper towel to prevent cracking.

Drizzle with second amount of salsa and sprinkle with cheese. Cover. Bake in 350°F (175°C) oven for 15 to 20 minutes until hot. Makes 12 enchiladas.

1 enchilada: 201 Calories; 5.4 g Total Fat (1.7 g Sat., 15.8 mg Cholesterol); 814 mg Sodium; 11 g Protein; 28 g Carbohydrate; 3 g Dietary Fibre

CHOICES: 1 1/2 Grains & Starches; 1 Meat & Alternatives

Fish Cakes

Serve with Tzatziki, page 116, or Roasted Red Pepper Sauce, page 117.

Cod (or snapper) fillets	3/4 lb.	340 g
Skim milk	1/3 cup	75 mL
Bay leaf	1	1
Medium potatoes, peeled and cut into small chunks (about 3/4 lb., 340 g)	2	2
Water	1/2 cup	125 mL
Salt	1/2 tsp.	2 mL
Non-fat plain yogurt	3 tbsp.	50 mL
Egg whites (large), fork-beaten	2	2
Dijon mustard	1 tbsp.	15 mL
Worcestershire sauce	1 tsp.	5 mL
Green onions, finely sliced	2	2
Salt	1/4 tsp.	1 mL
Pepper	1/8 tsp.	0.5 mL
Dill weed	1/2 tsp.	2 mL
Parsley flakes	1/2 tsp.	2 mL
Fine dry bread crumbs	2/3 cup	150 mL

Put first 3 ingredients into large non-stick frying pan. Cover. Poach on medium for 3 to 4 minutes until fish is opaque and flakes easily. Drain well. Remove and discard bay leaf. Chill fish.

Put next 3 ingredients into small saucepan. Cover. Bring to a boil. Heat for 15 minutes until soft. Drain, reserving about 1/4 cup (60 mL) water. Mash until no lumps remain.

Combine next 9 ingredients in small bowl. Add to potato. Mix well. Add fish. Stir, flaking fish with fork. Form into 10 patties.

Place bread crumbs on sheet of waxed paper. Coat each patty. Place on greased baking sheet. Spray patties well with cooking spray. Bake, uncovered, in 375°F (190°C) oven for 20 minutes until firm, golden brown and crisp. Makes 10 patties.

1 patty: 92 Calories; 0.7 g Total Fat (0.2 g Sat., 14.9 mg Cholesterol); 190 mg Sodium; 9 g Protein; 12 g Carbohydrate; 1 g Dietary Fibre

CHOICES: 1 Grains & Starches; 1 Meat & Alternatives

EASY FISH CAKES: Omit cod, milk and bay leaf. Use two 7 1/2 oz. (213 g) cans of salmon, drained and skin and round bones removed. Omit potatoes and first amount of salt. Use 1 1/2 cups (375 mL) leftover mashed potatoes.

Main Dishes

Vegetable Chili

Tastes even better the next day or after being frozen.
Keep small portions in the freezer to take for lunch.

Medium onion, chopped	1	1
Garlic cloves, minced (optional)	2	2
Chopped celery	1 cup	250 mL
Canola oil	2 tsp.	10 mL
Large red pepper, chopped	1/2	1/2
Large yellow pepper, chopped	1/2	1/2
Medium carrots, diced	2	2
Sliced fresh mushrooms	2 cups	500 mL
Diced medium zucchini, with peel	2 cups	500 mL
Can of diced tomatoes, with juice	14 oz.	398 mL
Can of red kidney beans, drained and rinsed	19 oz.	540 mL
Can of chick peas (garbanzo beans), drained and rinsed	19 oz.	540 mL
Can of beans in tomato sauce	14 oz.	398 mL
Chopped fresh parsley	1/4 cup	60 mL
Chili powder	2 tsp.	10 mL
Ground cumin (optional)	1/2 tsp.	2 mL
Dried whole oregano	1/2 tsp.	2 mL
Freshly ground pepper, sprinkle		
Dried crushed chilies (optional)	1/8 tsp.	0.5 mL
Bay leaf	1	1

Freshly ground pepper, for garnish

Sauté first 3 ingredients in canola oil in heavy-bottomed Dutch oven, stirring occasionally, until very soft.

Add next 16 ingredients. Cover. Simmer for about 1 1/2 hours until carrot is tender. Stir occasionally to prevent scorching.

Remove and discard bay leaf. Sprinkle with pepper. Makes 10 cups (2.5 L).

1 cup (250 mL): 179 Calories; 2.2 g Total Fat (0.2 g Sat., 0 mg Cholesterol); 484 mg Sodium; 9 g Protein; 34 g Carbohydrate; 9 g Dietary Fibre

CHOICES: 1 1/2 Grains & Starches; 1 Vegetables; 1 Meat & Alternatives

Pictured on page 107.

Bean Dumplings In Tomato Sauce

These dumplings provide a filling, nutritious meal with a different taste.

Chopped onion	1/2 cup	125 mL
Garlic cloves, minced	2	2
Chopped green pepper	1/2 cup	125 mL
Olive oil	2 tsp.	10 mL
Can of diced tomatoes, with juice	28 oz.	796 mL
Can of tomato juice	10 oz.	284 mL
Granulated sugar	1 1/2 tsp.	7 mL
Chili powder	1/2 tsp.	2 mL
Hot pepper sauce	1/4 tsp.	1 mL
All-purpose flour	2/3 cup	150 mL
Whole wheat flour	2/3 cup	150 mL
Baking powder	1 tbsp.	15 mL
Salt	1/4 tsp.	1 mL
Freshly ground pepper	1/8 tsp.	0.5 mL
Water	1/2 cup	125 mL
Can of white kidney beans, drained and rinsed	19 oz.	540 mL
Canola oil	2 tbsp.	30 mL
Egg whites (large)	2	2
Chopped green onion	1/2 cup	125 mL
Canola oil	1 tsp.	5 mL

Sauté first 3 ingredients in olive oil in large non-stick frying pan until onion is soft. Add next 5 ingredients. Bring to a boil. Simmer, uncovered, on medium for 30 minutes, stirring several times, until thickened.

Combine next 5 ingredients in medium bowl.

Process next 4 ingredients in food processor until almost smooth. Stir in green onion. Add to flour mixture. Stir just until moistened.

Divide and roll dough into about 50 balls (1/2 tbsp., 7 mL, each). Brown in canola oil in large non-stick frying pan. Add to sauce. Heat for 5 minutes until hot. Serves 6.

1 serving: 277 Calories; 8 g Total Fat (0.8 g Sat., 0 mg Cholesterol); 636 mg Sodium; 10 g Protein; 44 g Carbohydrate; 5 g Dietary Fibre

CHOICES: 2 Grains & Starches; 2 Vegetables; 1/2 Meat & Alternatives; 1 Fats

Pictured on page 107.

Spicy Rice And Beans

Quick and easy! Leave out the jalapeño pepper to tame the spicy heat.

Chopped onion	1 cup	250 mL
Garlic cloves, minced	3	3
Chopped celery	1/2 cup	125 mL
Jalapeño pepper, ribs and seeds removed, finely diced (see Tip, below)	1	1
Canola oil	1 tbsp.	15 mL
Ground cumin	1 tsp.	5 mL
Ground coriander	1 tsp.	5 mL
Chili powder	2 tsp.	10 mL
Long grain brown rice, uncooked	1 1/2 cups	375 mL
Grated carrot	1/2 cup	125 mL
Water	2 3/4 cups	675 mL
Vegetable bouillon powder	1 tbsp.	15 mL
Bay leaf	1	1
Can of red kidney beans, drained and rinsed	14 oz.	398 mL
Chopped tomato	1 cup	250 mL
Kernel corn, fresh or frozen	1/2 cup	125 mL
Chopped fresh cilantro (optional)	1 tbsp.	15 mL
Chopped fresh parsley (or 2 tsp., 10 mL, flakes)	2 tbsp.	30 mL

Sauté first 4 ingredients in canola oil in large non-stick frying pan for 3 minutes, stirring occasionally. Add next 4 ingredients. Cook on medium, stirring occasionally, until golden.

Stir in next 4 ingredients. Cover. Simmer on medium-low for 20 minutes.

Stir in next 3 ingredients. Cover. Heat for 15 to 20 minutes until liquid is absorbed. Remove and discard bay leaf.

Stir in cilantro and 1 tbsp. (15 mL) parsley. Garnish with remaining parsley. Makes 7 cups (1.75 L).

1 cup (250 mL): 253 Calories; 4 g Total Fat (0.5 g Sat., 0.2 mg Cholesterol); 356 mg Sodium; 8 g Protein; 48 g Carbohydrate; 5 g Dietary Fibre

CHOICES: 2 1/2 Grains & Starches; 1 Vegetables; 1/2 Fats

Pictured on page 107.

 tip   Hot peppers contain capsaicin in the seeds and ribs. Removing the seeds and ribs will lower the heat but wear rubber gloves when handling the peppers and avoid touching your eyes. Wash your hands well afterwards.

Chicken Supreme

Lots of sauce to flavour rice or noodles.

SAUCE		
Cold water	1 cup	250 mL
Cornstarch	2 tbsp.	30 mL
Low-sodium soy sauce	3 tbsp.	50 mL
Hoisin sauce	2 tbsp.	30 mL
Dried crushed chilies	1/2 tsp.	2 mL
Onion powder	1/2 tsp.	2 mL
Canola oil	2 tsp.	10 mL
Boneless, skinless chicken breast halves (about 3), cut into bite-size pieces	3/4 lb.	340 g
Canola oil	1 tsp.	5 mL
Thinly sliced mixed vegetables (such as carrots, celery, broccoli, cauliflower and green peppers)	6 cups	1.5 L
Medium onion, peeled and cut lengthwise into wedges	1	1
Garlic cloves, minced	2	2

Sauce: Combine first 6 ingredients in small bowl. Set aside. Makes about 1 1/2 cups (375 mL) sauce.

Heat first amount of canola oil in non-stick frying pan or wok on medium-high. Add chicken. Stir-fry for about 4 minutes until no pink remains in chicken. Remove to bowl.

Heat second amount of canola oil in same frying pan or wok. Stir-fry next 3 ingredients for about 8 minutes until tender-crisp. Add chicken. Stir sauce. Add to chicken mixture. Heat and stir until boiling and thickened. Makes 6 cups (1.5 L).

1 cup (250 mL): 147 Calories; 3.4 g Total Fat (0.4 g Sat., 32.9 mg Cholesterol); 889 mg Sodium; 16 g Protein; 14 g Carbohydrate; 3 g Dietary Fibre

CHOICES: 3 Vegetables; 2 Meat & Alternatives

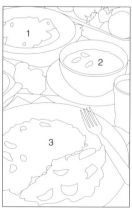

1. Bean Dumplings In Tomato Sauce, page 104
2. Vegetable Chili, page 103
3. Spicy Rice And Beans, page 105

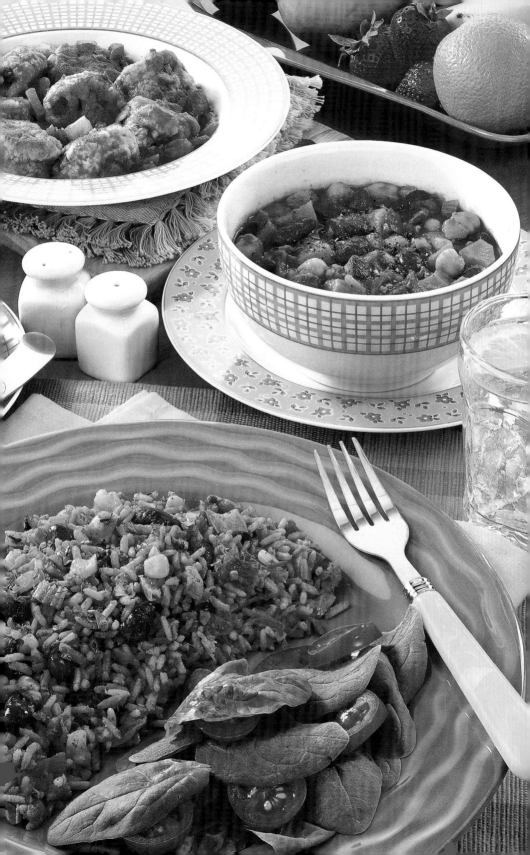

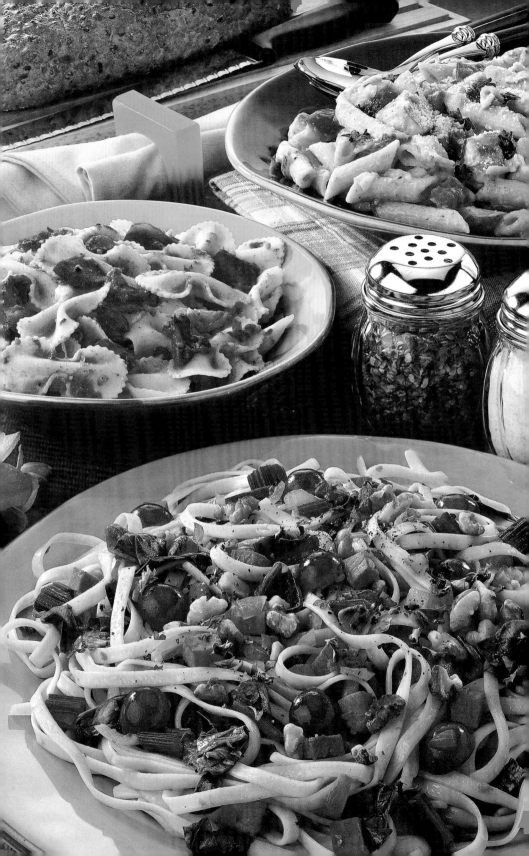

Grilled Hoisin Flank Steak

Marinade is reduced and doubles as a flavourful baste.

Low-sodium soy sauce	3 tbsp.	50 mL
Hoisin sauce	3 tbsp.	50 mL
Water	1/2 cup	125 mL
Green onion	1	1
Hot chili paste	1/2 tsp.	2 mL
Garlic cloves	3	3
Slice of peeled gingerroot (1/4 inch 6 mm, length)	1/2	1/2
Dry red (or alcohol-free) wine	1/4 cup	60 mL
Lemon juice	2 tbsp.	30 mL
Flank steak, trimmed and scored on both sides	1 1/2 lbs.	680 g

Put first 9 ingredients into blender. Blend until smooth. Pour into large sealable freezer bag. Add steak. Seal. Chill for several hours or overnight, turning several times. Drain marinade into small saucepan. Bring to a boil. Heat until reduced by half and slightly thickened. Makes 1/2 cup (125 mL) sauce. Grill steak over medium-high heat on barbecue for about 5 minutes per side, basting several times with sauce, until desired doneness. Thinly slice across grain at slight angle. Discard any remaining sauce. Serves 6.

1 serving: 219 Calories; 8.4 g Total Fat (3.6 g Sat., 46.1 mg Cholesterol); 747 mg Sodium; 26 g Protein; 7 g Carbohydrate; trace Dietary Fibre

CHOICES: 3 1/2 Meat & Alternatives

Pictured on page 72.

Variation: Grill steak on medium-high in indoor double-sided grill. Heat for about 10 minutes, basting several times, until desired doneness.

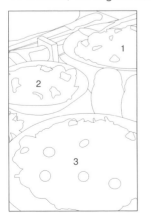

1. Creamy Garlic Penne, page 110
2. Roasted Pepper And Tomato Pasta, page 113
3. Red Chard And Garlic Pasta, page 111

Creamy Garlic Penne

For garlic lovers only! Nice bite from the cayenne pepper.

Can of skim evaporated milk	13 1/2 oz.	385 mL
Skim milk	1 1/3 cups	325 mL
All-purpose flour	3 tbsp.	50 mL
Garlic cloves, minced	2 – 4	2 – 4
Vegetable bouillon powder	2 tsp.	10 mL
Boneless, skinless chicken breast halves (about 3), cut into bite-size pieces	3/4 lb.	340 g
Olive oil	2 tsp.	10 mL
Cayenne pepper	1/2 tsp.	2 mL
Coarsely ground pepper	1/4 tsp.	1 mL
Chopped fresh tomato	1 cup	250 mL
Imitation crabmeat (about 6 oz., 170 g)	1 1/2 cups	375 mL
Penne pasta (10 oz., 285 g)	3 cups	750 mL
Boiling water	2 qts.	2 L
Salt (optional)	1 tbsp.	15 mL
Grated light Parmesan cheese (optional)	2 tbsp.	30 mL
Chopped fresh parsley (optional)		

Whisk both milks into flour in large non-stick frying pan until smooth. Add garlic and bouillon powder. Heat and stir on medium-low until boiling and thickened. Keep warm on low, stirring occasionally.

Sauté chicken in olive oil in non-stick frying pan for 5 minutes until slightly browned. Sprinkle with cayenne and pepper. Add tomato and crabmeat. Toss well until hot. Add to milk mixture. Stir. Keep warm.

Cook pasta in boiling water and salt in large pot or Dutch oven for 10 to 12 minutes until just tender. Drain.

Turn pasta into serving dish. Pour sauce over top. Toss to coat. Sprinkle with Parmesan cheese and parsley. Makes 7 1/2 cups (1.9 L). Serves 6.

1 serving: 379 Calories; 3.9 g Total Fat (0.8 g Sat., 46.7 mg Cholesterol); 549 mg Sodium; 31 g Protein; 54 g Carbohydrate; 2 g Dietary Fibre

CHOICES: 2 1/2 Grains & Starches; 1 Milk & Alternatives; 2 Meat & Alternatives

Pictured on page 108.

Red Chard And Garlic Pasta

A very different combination of flavours, and they go together so well.

Finely chopped onion	1 cup	250 mL
Garlic cloves, minced	5	5
Olive oil	2 tsp.	10 mL
Red chard (1 bunch)	1 lb.	454 g
Water	1/4 cup	60 mL
Vegetable bouillon powder	1 tsp.	5 mL
Finely diced non-fat, low-sodium ham	1/2 cup	125 mL
Balsamic vinegar	2 tbsp.	30 mL
Seedless red grapes, halved	30	30
Fettuccine	12 oz.	340 g
Boiling water	3 qts.	3 L
Salt	1 tbsp.	15 mL
Chopped walnuts, toasted (see Tip, below)	1/3 cup	75 mL
Chopped fresh parsley	1/4 cup	60 mL

Sauté onion and garlic in olive oil in large non-stick frying pan until onion is soft.

Fold each chard leaf lengthwise along the rib. Cut ribs out. Slice ribs crosswise. Coarsely chop leaves and set aside. Add ribs and next 3 ingredients to onion and garlic. Cover. Heat for 5 minutes until chard ribs are tender. Stir in vinegar and grapes. Keep warm.

Cook pasta in boiling water and salt in large uncovered pot or Dutch oven for 10 minutes. Stir in chard leaves. Cook for 2 to 3 minutes until pasta is tender but firm. Drain. Return to pot.

Add chard ribs mixture. Toss. Garnish with walnuts and parsley. Makes 8 cups (2 L). Serves 6.

1 1/2 cups (375 mL): 321 Calories; 7.3 g Total Fat (0.8 g Sat., 0.1 mg Cholesterol); 424 mg Sodium; 12 g Protein; 53 g Carbohydrate; 4 g Dietary Fibre

CHOICES: 3 Grains & Starches; 1 Vegetables; 1 Fats

Pictured on page 108.

 tip To toast nuts or coconut, place in shallow pan. Bake in 350°F (175°C) oven for 5 to 10 minutes, stirring often, until desired doneness.

Salmon Rice Mélange

Make rice the night before, and this casserole goes together in minutes.

Package of long grain and wild rice mix	6 1/4 oz.	180 g
Chopped onion	1/2 cup	125 mL
Chopped celery	1/2 cup	125 mL
Canola oil	2 tsp.	10 mL
All-purpose flour	2 tbsp.	30 mL
No-salt herb seasoning	1/2 tsp.	2 mL
Skim evaporated milk	3/4 cup	175 mL
Skim milk	3/4 cup	175 mL
Low-sodium soy sauce	1 tbsp.	15 mL
Frozen peas	1 cup	250 mL
Can of red salmon, drained, skin and round bones removed	7 1/2 oz.	213 g
Fine dry bread crumbs	1/4 cup	60 mL
Grated light Monterey Jack cheese	1/2 cup	125 mL

Cook rice mix as per package directions without margarine.

Saute onion and celery in canola oil in non-stick frying pan for 5 minutes until soft. Sprinkle flour and herb seasoning over top. Stir for 1 minute. Slowly add both milks, stirring constantly, until smooth.

Stir in soy sauce and peas until boiling and thickened. Add rice and salmon. Stir gently. Turn into greased 1 1/2 quart (1.5 L) casserole.

Combine bread crumbs and cheese. Sprinkle over top. Bake, uncovered, in 350°F (175°C) oven for 20 to 30 minutes until edges are bubbling and casserole is hot in center. Serves 6.

1 serving: 457 Calories; 7.2 g Total Fat (2.7 g Sat., 23.6 mg Cholesterol); 633 mg Sodium; 19 g Protein; 40 g Carbohydrate; 2 g Dietary Fibre

CHOICES: 2 Grains & Starches; 1/2 Milk & Alternatives; 2 Meat & Alternatives; 1/2 Fats

Chicken Chili

Serve on brown rice or as is with salad. Uses Tomato Vegetable Sauce, page 118.

Lean ground chicken	3/4 lb.	340 g
Finely chopped celery	1/2 cup	125 mL
Container of Tomato Vegetable Sauce (3 cups, 750 mL), page 118, thawed	1	1
Chili powder	2 tsp.	10 mL
Can of red kidney beans, drained and rinsed	14 oz.	398 mL

(continued on next page)

Scramble-fry ground chicken and celery in non-stick frying pan until starting to brown. Drain. Add remaining 3 ingredients. Cover. Simmer for 30 minutes to blend flavours. Makes 5 cups (1.25 L).

1 1/4 cups (300 mL): 239 Calories; 3.1 g Total Fat (0.5 g Sat., 49.3 mg Cholesterol); 472 mg Sodium; 27 g Protein; 27 g Carbohydrate; 8 g Dietary Fibre

CHOICES: 1/2 Grains & Starches; 2 1/2 Vegetables; 3 1/2 Meat & Alternatives

---

Roasted Pepper And Tomato Pasta

You can't beat this for easy—and the flavour is sublime!

Medium red peppers, cut into 1 inch (2.5 cm) pieces (about 4 cups, 1 L)	3	3
Medium Roma (plum) tomatoes, diced (about 4 cups, 1 L)	8	8
Garlic cloves, halved	8	8
Olive oil	1 tbsp.	15 mL
Granulated sugar, pinch		
Salt	1/4 tsp.	1 mL
Freshly ground pepper, sprinkle		
Medium bow (or shell) pasta (about 10 oz., 285 g)	3 cups	750 mL
Boiling water	3 qts.	3 L
Salt	1 tbsp.	15 mL
Grated light Parmesan cheese	3 tbsp.	50 mL

Combine first 3 ingredients in large greased shallow glass casserole or enameled roaster (see Note). Drizzle with olive oil. Toss to coat. Bake in 425°F (220°C) oven for 30 minutes. Mix. Bake for 40 minutes until pepper is soft. Sprinkle with next 3 ingredients. Mash slightly with fork.

Cook pasta in water and salt in large uncovered pot or Dutch oven for 10 minutes until tender but firm. Drain.

Toss pasta, tomato mixture and Parmesan cheese. Serves 4.

1 serving: 384 Calories; 6.2 g Total Fat (1.2 g Sat., 1.9 mg Cholesterol); 283 mg Sodium; 14 g Protein; 70 g Carbohydrate; 6 g Dietary Fibre

CHOICES: 3 1/2 Grains & Starches; 3 Vegetables; 1/2 Meat & Alternatives; 1 Fats

Pictured on page 108.

Note: Don't cook tomatoes in a metal pan as taste can be altered by a reaction of the acid and metal.

Beef And Sprout Stir-Fry

Crunchy with lots of sauce to serve on noodles or rice.

SAUCE		
Water	1/2 cup	125 mL
Cornstarch	1 tbsp.	15 mL
Low-sodium soy sauce	1/4 cup	60 mL
Garlic powder (optional)	1/8 tsp.	0.5 mL
Canola oil	2 tsp.	10 mL
Lean sirloin steak, trimmed and cut crosswise into very thin slices	3/4 lb.	340 g
Garlic cloves, minced	2	2
Sliced fresh mushrooms	1 cup	250 mL
Thinly sliced celery	1/2 cup	125 mL
Coarsely shredded carrot	1/2 cup	125 mL
Chopped green onion	1/2 cup	125 mL
Fresh bean sprouts	3 cups	750 mL

Sauce: Stir first 4 ingredients in small bowl. Set aside. Makes about 7/8 cup (200 mL) sauce.

Heat canola oil in non-stick frying pan or wok on medium-high. Add beef and garlic. Stir-fry for 3 minutes. Add next 3 ingredients. Stir-fry for 4 minutes.

Stir sauce. Add to beef mixture. Add green onion and bean sprouts. Heat and stir for 2 minutes until boiling and thickened. Makes 4 cups (1 L).

1 cup (250 mL): 213 Calories; 8.9 g Total Fat (2.9 g Sat., 34.6 mg Cholesterol); 736 mg Sodium; 23 g Protein; 11 g Carbohydrate; 2 g Dietary Fibre

CHOICES: 2 Vegetables; 3 Meat & Alternatives; 1/2 Fats

Green Pepper Beef Loaf

A delicious dinner that's also great for sandwiches the next day.

Medium green pepper, cut into chunks	1	1
Skim evaporated milk	1/2 cup	125 mL
Large egg	1	1
Chopped onion	1/4 cup	60 mL
Onion salt	1 tsp.	5 mL
Freshly ground pepper, sprinkle		
Parsley flakes	1 tsp.	5 mL
Extra lean ground beef	1 1/2 lbs.	680 g
Fine dry bread crumbs	1/2 cup	125 mL

(continued on next page)

Main Dishes

Process first 7 ingredients in blender until pepper and onion are quite finely chopped. Pour into medium bowl.

Add ground beef and bread crumbs. Mix very well. Pack into foil-lined, greased 9 x 5 x 3 inch (22 x 12.5 x 7.5 cm) loaf pan. Bake, uncovered, in 350°F (175°C) oven for 1 1/2 to 2 hours until no pink remains in beef. Drain off liquid. Turn out onto plate. Peel off foil. Cuts into 10 slices.

1 slice: 212 Calories; 10.2 g Total Fat (3.9 g Sat., 76.9 mg Cholesterol); 256 mg Sodium; 22 g Protein; 7 g Carbohydrate; trace Dietary Fibre

CHOICES: 1/2 Grains & Starches; 3 Meat & Alternatives;

Vegetable Gravy

This versatile sauce can be used as a stroganoff sauce for beef or chicken just by adding a little non-fat or light sour cream. Also good as a sauce for meatballs. Make a double batch of base and freeze to always have on hand.

Water	3 cups	750 mL
Vegetable bouillon powder	1 tbsp.	15 mL
Garlic cloves, peeled	8	8
Large carrot, cut into 1 inch (2.5 cm) pieces	1	1
Large celery rib, cut into 1 inch (2.5 cm) pieces	1	1
Large onion, chopped	1	1
Cornstarch (see Note)	2 tbsp.	30 mL
Water	1/4 cup	60 mL
Light sour cream (optional)	1/4 cup	60 mL

Bring water to a boil in large saucepan. Add next 5 ingredients. Cover. Simmer for about 40 minutes until vegetables are very soft. Blend in saucepan with hand blender. Freeze at this point if desired.

Stir water into cornstarch in small dish. Stir into vegetable mixture. Heat and stir on medium, until boiling and slightly thickened. Stir in sour cream. Makes 4 cups (1 L).

1/2 cup (125 mL): 29 Calories; 0.2 g Total Fat (0.1 g Sat., 0.1 mg Cholesterol); 234 mg Sodium; 1 g Protein; 6 g Carbohydrate; 1 g Dietary Fibre

CHOICES: 1 Vegetables

Note: To freeze, omit cornstarch and water. Freeze in 2 cup (500 mL) portions. After thawing, thicken with 1 tbsp. (15 mL) cornstarch and 2 tbsp. (30 mL) water.

Creamy Pasta Sauce

Serve this garlicky sauce on your favourite pasta.

Garlic cloves, minced	4	4
Olive oil	2 tsp.	10 mL
Can of skim evaporated milk	13 1/2 oz.	385 mL
All-purpose flour	2 tbsp.	30 mL
Container of Tomato Vegetable Sauce (3 cups, 750 mL), page 118, thawed	1	1
Dried sweet basil	1/2 tsp.	2 mL
Dried whole oregano	1/2 tsp.	2 mL
Salt	1/4 tsp.	1 mL
Pepper	1/8 tsp.	0.5 mL

Sauté garlic in olive oil in medium saucepan until soft.

Whisk evaporated milk into flour in small bowl. Add to saucepan. Heat, stirring constantly, until boiling and thickened.

Add next 3 ingredients. Heat and stir until heated through. Add salt and pepper. Stir. Makes 4 cups (1 L).

1/2 cup (125 mL): 95 Calories; 2.1 g Total Fat (0.3 g Sat., 1.9 mg Cholesterol); 273 mg Sodium; 6 g Protein; 14 g Carbohydrate; 2 g Dietary Fibre

CHOICES: 1 Vegetables; 1/2 Milk & Alternatives; 1/2 Fats

Variation: For a smooth sauce, purée in blender to desired consistency.

Tzatziki

Always a favourite and so healthy when using non-fat Yogurt Cheese, page 75.
Serve on warmed and torn pita bread or with Fish Cakes, page 102.

Grated English cucumber, with peel	1 cup	250 mL
Salt	1 1/2 tsp.	7 mL
Yogurt Cheese, page 75	1 cup	250 mL
Granulated sugar	1/4 tsp.	1 mL
Garlic clove(s), minced	1 – 2	1 – 2
Salt	1/4 tsp.	1 mL
Freshly ground pepper, sprinkle		

(continued on next page)

Place cucumber in colander over small bowl. Sprinkle with salt. Let stand in refrigerator for 2 hours. Squeeze out excess moisture. Discard liquid. Empty cucumber into medium bowl.

Stir in remaining 5 ingredients. Cover. Chill for 1 to 2 hours to blend flavours. Makes 1 1/2 cups (375 mL).

1 tbsp. (15 mL): 12 Calories; 0.3 g Total Fat (0.2 g Sat., 1.1 mg Cholesterol); 121 mg Sodium; 1 g Protein; 1 g Carbohydrate; trace Dietary Fibre

CHOICES: None

Roasted Red Pepper Sauce

Try this on Fish Cakes, page 102, poached fish fillets or in a sandwich wrap. Will keep covered in refrigerator for up to one week.

Frozen egg product, thawed (see Note)	1/2 cup	125 mL
Garlic cloves	2	2
Non-fat mayonnaise (not salad dressing)	1/2 cup	125 mL
Lemon juice	2 tsp.	10 mL
Salt	1/8 tsp.	0.5 mL
Cayenne pepper, sprinkle		
Olive oil, heated to 250° – 300°F (120° – 150°C)	1/3 cup	75 mL
Can of roasted red peppers, drained and blotted dry, cut into strips	14 oz.	398 mL

Process egg substitute and garlic in blender until garlic is finely chopped. Add next 4 ingredients. Process, scraping down sides if necessary, until smooth.

With blender running, slowly and carefully add hot olive oil in steady stream through hole in lid.

With blender running, add red pepper strips, 1 at a time, allowing each piece to completely blend before adding another, periodically scraping down sides. Makes 2 cups (500 mL).

2 tbsp. (30 mL): 52 Calories; 4.6 g Total Fat (0.6 g Sat., 0 mg Cholesterol); 82 mg Sodium; 1 g Protein; 2 g Carbohydrate; trace Dietary Fibre

CHOICES: 1 Fats

Note: 4 tbsp. (50 mL) = 1 large egg

Tomato Vegetable Sauce

Serve on pasta as is or freeze in batches and then use in
Chicken Chili, page 112, Creamy Pasta Sauce, page 116,
Cheese Spirals, page 131, or Minestrone Soup, page 153.

Chopped onion	2 cups	500 mL
Garlic cloves, minced	6	6
Olive oil	1 tbsp.	15 mL
Cans of diced tomatoes (28 oz., 796 mL, each), with juice	3	3
Can of tomato paste	5 1/2 oz.	156 mL
Zucchini, quartered lengthwise and sliced	4 cups	1 L
Medium green, red or yellow peppers, chopped	3	3
Dried sweet basil	2 tsp.	10 mL
Dried whole oregano	2 tsp.	10 mL
Parsley flakes	2 tsp.	10 mL
Coarsely ground pepper	1/2 tsp.	2 mL
Bay leaf	1	1
Granulated sugar	1 tsp.	5 mL

Sauté onion and garlic in olive oil in large non-stick frying pan, stirring frequently, until onion is golden. Turn into 4 quart (4 L) casserole or small roaster.

Stir in remaining 10 ingredients. Bake, uncovered, in 350°F (175°C) oven for 3 hours, stirring occasionally, until slightly thickened. Remove and discard bay leaf. Mash mixture slightly. Makes 12 cups (3 L). Divide into four 3 cup (750 mL) freezer containers. Label. Freeze.

1/2 cup (125 mL): 45 Calories; 1 g Total Fat (0.1 g Sat., 0 mg Cholesterol); 171 mg Sodium; 2 g Protein; 9 g Carbohydrate; 2 g Dietary Fibre

CHOICES: 1 1/2 Vegetables

Paré Pointer
They threw eggs at the actor because ham and eggs go together.

Mediterranean Garbanzo Salad

All the flavours come together in a full and rich taste once salad has chilled.

Can of garbanzo beans (chick peas), drained and rinsed	19 oz.	540 g
Diced English cucumber, with peel	1 cup	250 mL
Medium Roma (plum) tomatoes, seeded and diced (about 1 1/3 cups, 325 mL)	3	3
Finely chopped red onion	1/4 cup	60 mL
Diced green pepper	1/2 cup	125 mL
Sliced ripe olives	1/4 cup	60 mL
FETA CHEESE DRESSING		
1% buttermilk	2 tbsp.	30 mL
Olive oil	1 tsp.	5 mL
Chopped fresh oregano leaves (or 1 tsp., 5 mL, dried)	2 tsp.	10 mL
Chopped fresh parsley (or 2 tsp., 10 mL, flakes)	1 tbsp.	15 mL
Light feta cheese, crumbled	1/2 cup	125 mL
Freshly ground pepper, sprinkle		
Grated lemon peel (or juice)	1 tsp.	5 mL
Garlic clove(s), minced (or 1/4 tsp., 1 mL, powder)	1	1

Combine first 6 ingredients in large bowl. Makes 6 cups (1.5 L) vegetables.

Feta Cheese Dressing: Process all 8 ingredients in blender until quite smooth. Makes 2/3 cup (150 mL) dressing. Add to vegetables. Toss to coat. Chill for at least 1 to 2 hours to blend flavours. Serves 8.

1 serving: 99 Calories; 3.8 g Total Fat (1.6 g Sat., 8.3 mg Cholesterol); 208 mg Sodium; 5 g Protein; 13 g Carbohydrate; 2 g Dietary Fibre

CHOICES: 1/2 Grains & Starches; 1/2 Vegetables; 1/2 Meat & Alternatives; 1/2 Fats

Pictured on page 125.

Quick Pasta Salad

Using canned peppers and enhancing bottled dressing makes this fast to prepare.

Rotini pasta	2 cups	500 mL
Boiling water	2 qts.	2 L
Salt	2 tsp.	10 mL
Can of roasted red peppers, drained and cut into 2 inch (5 cm) slivers	14 oz.	398 mL
Paper-thin sliced red onion	1 cup	250 mL
Non-fat French dressing	1/2 cup	125 mL
Garlic clove(s), minced	1 – 2	1 – 2
Dried whole oregano, crushed	1/4 tsp.	1 mL
Freshly ground pepper, sprinkle		

Cook pasta in boiling water and salt in large uncovered saucepan for 10 to 12 minutes until tender but firm. Drain. Rinse well with cold water. Drain.

Combine pasta with red pepper and onion in medium bowl.

Combine remaining 4 ingredients in small bowl. Pour over salad. Mix well. Cover. Chill. Serves 4.

1 serving: 248 Calories; 0.9 g Total Fat (0.1 g Sat., 0 mg Cholesterol); 444 mg Sodium; 8 g Protein; 52 g Carbohydrate; 4 g Dietary Fibre

CHOICES: 2 Grains & Starches; 2 Vegetables;

Cheese And Artichoke Salad

The perfect recipe for a time crunch—only 15 minutes preparation time!

DRESSING

Non-fat Italian dressing	1/2 cup	125 mL
White (or alcohol-free) wine	2 tbsp.	30 mL
Small garlic clove, minced	1	1
Dried rosemary (or pinch of ground rosemary)	1/2 tsp.	2 mL
Large shell pasta (not jumbo), about 5 oz. (140 g)	1 3/4 cups	425 mL
Boiling water	6 cups	1.5 L
Salt	1 1/2 tsp.	7 mL
Can of artichoke hearts, drained and chopped	14 oz.	398 mL
Part-skim mozzarella cheese, cut into 1/2 inch (12 mm) cubes	4 oz.	113 g
Diced red pepper	1/4 cup	60 mL

(continued on next page)

Salads

Dressing: Combine first 4 ingredients in small bowl. Let stand at room temperature for at least 15 minutes. Makes about 2/3 cup (150 mL) dressing.

Cook pasta in boiling water and salt in large saucepan for about 8 minutes until tender but firm. Drain. Rinse with cold water. Drain. Place in medium bowl.

Add remaining 3 ingredients. Add dressing. Toss to coat. Cover. Chill. Makes 5 cups (1.25 L).

1 cup (250 mL): 200 Calories; 4.3 g Total Fat (2.4 g Sat., 13.5 mg Cholesterol); 536 mg Sodium; 11 g Protein; 29 g Carbohydrate; 3 g Dietary Fibre

CHOICES: 1 1/2 Grains & Starches; 1 Meat & Alternatives

Marinated Salad

You'll love the refreshing combination of the vegetables and marinade. So easy to make ahead. The bulgur makes it chewy.

Bulgur wheat	1/2 cup	125 mL
Boiling water	1 1/2 cups	375 mL
Seeded, diced tomato	2 cups	500 mL
Diced English cucumber, with peel	2 cups	500 mL
Diced green pepper	1 cup	250 mL
Sliced ripe olives	1/2 cup	125 mL
Thinly sliced green onion	1/4 cup	60 mL
Feta cheese, crumbled into small pieces, (optional)	3/4 cup	175 mL
Olive oil	2 tbsp.	30 mL
Lemon juice	2 tbsp.	30 mL
Dried whole oregano, crushed	1/4 tsp.	1 mL
Salt	1/4 tsp.	1 mL
Freshly ground pepper, to taste		
Torn romaine lettuce	6 cups	1.5 L

Soak bulgur in boiling water in small saucepan for 10 minutes. Drain. Set aside.

Combine next 11 ingredients in large bowl. Cover. Let stand at room temperature for 30 minutes. Drain and discard liquid. Add bulgur.

Add lettuce. Toss gently. Serve immediately. Serves 8.

1 serving: 70 Calories; 1.9 g Total Fat (0.3 g Sat., 0 mg Cholesterol); 142 mg Sodium; 3 g Protein; 12 g Carbohydrate; 4 g Dietary Fibre

CHOICES: 1/2 Grains & Starches; 1 Vegetables; 1/2 Fats

Pictured on front cover.

Vinaigrette Potato Salad

Double or triple the recipe to serve a crowd.

Unpeeled baby potatoes	1 lb.	454 g
Water		
Medium carrot, coarsely grated	1	1
Coarsely chopped red pepper	1 cup	250 mL
Green onions, sliced	2	2
DRESSING		
Vegetable bouillon powder	1 tsp.	5 mL
Hot water	1/4 cup	60 mL
Olive oil	2 tbsp.	30 mL
Balsamic vinegar	1 tbsp.	15 mL
Lemon juice	1 tbsp.	15 mL
Garlic clove	1	1
Chopped fresh parsley (or 1 tsp., 5 mL, flakes)	1 tbsp.	15 mL
Chopped fresh marjoram leaves (or 1 tsp., 5 mL, dried)	1 tbsp.	15 mL
Dijon mustard	1 tsp.	5 mL
Salt	1/2 tsp.	2 mL
Freshly ground pepper, sprinkle		

Cook potatoes in water in small saucepan until tender. Drain. Cool. Cut into quarters, or in halves if very small. Place in medium bowl.

Add next 3 ingredients to bowl.

Dressing: Dissolve bouillon powder in hot water in blender. Add remaining 9 ingredients. Process. Pour over salad. Toss. Chill. Toss before serving. Makes 4 cups (1 L).

1 cup (250 mL): 169 Calories; 7.3 g Total Fat (1.0 g Sat., 0.1 mg Cholesterol); 524 mg Sodium; 3 g Protein; 24 g Carbohydrate; 3 g Dietary Fibre

CHOICES: 1 Grains & Starches; 2 Vegetables; 1 1/2 Fats

Pictured on page 125.

 tip There is no need to cover potatoes with water while boiling. To cook potatoes without losing their nutrients, add 1/2 to 1 inch (1.2 to 2.5 cm) water to the pot. Cover. Bring to a boil. Reduce heat. Simmer until desired doneness.

Couscous Seafood Salad

Slightly chewy with just enough dressing to flavour.

Couscous	1/2 cup	125 mL
Boiling water	2/3 cup	150 mL
Finely diced green pepper	1/2 cup	125 mL
Finely diced celery	1/4 cup	60 mL
Thinly sliced green onion	2 tbsp.	30 mL
Chopped imitation crabmeat	3/4 cup	175 mL
(about 3 oz., 85 g)		
Frozen tiny peas, thawed	1/2 cup	125 mL
Shredded fresh spinach leaves	3/4 cup	175 mL
Toasted sesame seeds (see Tip, page 111)	2 tsp.	10 mL
DRESSING		
Rice vinegar	2 tbsp.	30 mL
Ketchup	2 tsp.	10 mL
Granulated sugar	1/2 tsp.	2 mL
Garlic powder	1/8 tsp.	0.5 mL
Ground coriander	1/16 tsp.	0.5 mL
Ground oregano	1/16 tsp.	0.5 mL
Canola oil	1 tsp.	5 mL

Stir couscous into boiling water. Cover. Let stand for 5 minutes. Fluff with fork. Turn into medium bowl. Cool.

Add next 7 ingredients. Toss.

Dressing: Whisk all 7 ingredients in small bowl. Pour over spinach mixture. Toss lightly. Makes 4 cups (1 L). Serves 4.

1 cup (250 mL): 161 Calories; 2.5 g Total Fat (0.4 g Sat., 7.7 mg Cholesterol); 225 mg Sodium; 8 g Protein; 27 g Carbohydrate; 3 g Dietary Fibre

CHOICES: 1 Grains & Starches; 2 Vegetables; 1/2 Meat & Alternatives;

Artichoke Salad

A delicious and nutritious salad with a colourful presentation.

Medium tomato, cut into 8 wedges	1	1
English cucumber slices, with peel	8	8
Medium ripe olives, cut in half	8	8
Can of artichoke hearts, drained and cut into quarters	14 oz.	398 mL
Medium green pepper, thinly sliced	1/2	1/2
Small red onion, thinly sliced	1/2	1/2
Olive oil	2 tbsp.	30 mL
Lemon juice	1 tbsp.	15 mL
White wine vinegar	1 1/2 tsp.	7 mL
Liquid honey	1 1/2 tsp.	7 mL
Garlic clove, minced	1	1
Dried whole oregano	1/4 tsp.	1 mL
Freshly ground pepper, sprinkle		
Mixed salad greens	6 cups	1.5 L
Crumbled feta cheese, optional	1/4 cup	60 mL

Combine first 6 ingredients in medium bowl.

Whisk next 7 ingredients together in small bowl. Pour onto vegetable mixture. Gently toss. Chill for at least 1 hour to blend flavours.

Arrange on bed of salad greens. Sprinkle with cheese. Serves 4.

1 serving: 138 Calories; 8.3 g Total Fat (1.1 g Sat., 0 mg Cholesterol); 280 mg Sodium; 4 g Protein; 15 g Carbohydrate; 5 g Dietary Fibre

CHOICES: 2 Vegetables; 1/2 Meat & Alternatives; 1 1/2 Fats

Pictured at right.

1. Mediterranean Garbanzo Salad, page 119
2. Fresh Strawberry Dressing, page 128
3. Creamy Orange Dressing, page 128
4. Artichoke Salad, above
5. Vinaigrette Potato Salad, page 122

Props courtesy of: Winners Stores

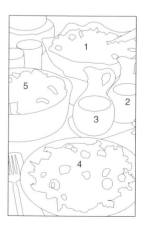

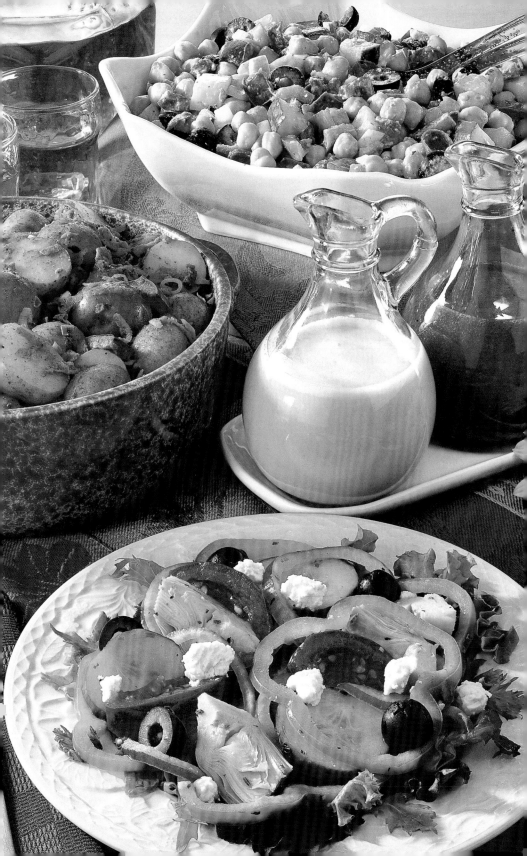

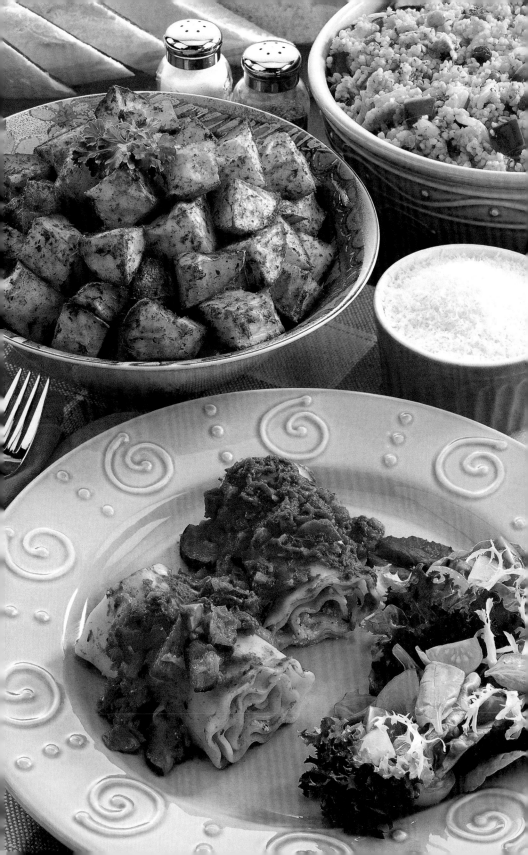

Caesar Salad Dressing

You'll never miss the eggs and oil in this tasty substitute for high-fat Caesar dressing.

Garlic clove(s)	1 – 2	1 – 2
Water	1 tbsp.	15 mL
Lemon juice	1 tbsp.	15 mL
Red wine vinegar	1 tbsp.	15 mL
Dry mustard	1/4 tsp.	1 mL
Silken (or soft) tofu	3/4 cup	175 mL
Anchovy paste	1 tbsp.	15 mL
Salt	1/8 tsp.	0.5 mL
Freshly ground pepper, sprinkle		
Grated light Parmesan cheese	1 tbsp.	15 mL

Process all 10 ingredients in blender until smooth. Makes 1 cup (250 mL).

2 tbsp. (30 mL): 27 Calories; 1.5 g Total Fat (0.3 g Sat., 2.4 mg Cholesterol); 150 mg Sodium; 3 g Protein; 1 g Carbohydrate; trace Dietary Fibre

CHOICES: 1/2 Meat & Alternatives

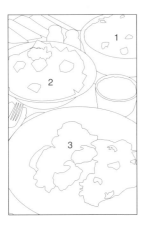

1. Bulgur Curry, page 145
2. Spicy Potato Bumps, page 130
3. Cheese Spirals, page 131

Creamy Orange Dressing

Serve this refreshing dressing with spinach or mixed salad greens.

Frozen concentrated orange juice, thawed (half of 12 1/2 oz., 355 mL, can)	3/4 cup	175 mL
White wine vinegar	2 tbsp.	30 mL
Non-fat plain yogurt	1/2 cup	125 mL
Liquid honey (or sugar substitute, such as Sugar Twin, to taste)	1 tbsp.	15 mL
Ground cinnamon	1/4 tsp.	1 mL

Whisk all 5 ingredients in small bowl until smooth. Makes 1 1/2 cups (375 mL).

2 tbsp. (30 mL): 40 Calories; 0.1 g Total Fat (trace Sat., 0.2 mg Cholesterol); 8 mg Sodium; 1 g Protein; 9 g Carbohydrate; trace Dietary Fibre

CHOICES: 1/2 Fruits

Pictured on page 125.

Fresh Strawberry Dressing

Wonderful strawberry flavour with a nice peppery aftertaste.

Chopped fresh strawberries	1 cup	250 mL
White wine vinegar	1 tbsp.	15 mL
Balsamic vinegar	1 1/2 tsp.	7 mL
Liquid honey (optional)	1 tsp.	5 mL
Freshly ground pepper	1 tsp.	5 mL

Process all 5 ingredients in blender until smooth. Makes 1 cup (250 mL).

2 tbsp. (30 mL): 6 Calories; 0.1 g Total Fat (trace Sat., 0 mg Cholesterol); trace Sodium; trace Protein; 2 g Carbohydrate; trace Dietary Fibre

CHOICES: None

Pictured on page 125.

Vegetable Medley

Put these in with a roast, and everything will be ready at the same time.

Red baby potatoes, halved	1 lb.	454 g
Medium sweet potatoes, cut bite size (about 1 lb., 454 g)	2	2
Parsnips, cut bite size (about 2 cups, 500 mL)	3	3
Carrots, cut bite size (about 2 1/2 cups, 625 mL)	5	5
Chopped onion	2/3 cup	150 mL
Boiling water	3 tbsp.	50 mL
Margarine	1 tsp.	5 mL
Chicken bouillon powder	1/2 tsp.	2 mL
Garlic clove(s), minced (optional)	1 – 2	1 – 2
Parsley flakes	1/2 tsp.	2 mL
Seasoned salt	1/2 tsp.	2 mL
Pepper	1/8 tsp.	0.5 mL

Place first 4 ingredients in greased 9 x 13 inch (22 x 33 cm) baking pan or shallow 2 quart (2 L) casserole. Add onion. Stir.

Pour boiling water over margarine and bouillon powder in small bowl. Stir to dissolve. Stir in remaining 4 ingredients. Pour bouillon mixture over vegetables. Toss gently. Cover tightly with foil or lid. Bake in 350°F (175°C) oven for 1 1/2 hours until vegetables are tender. Uncover for last 10 to 15 minutes to evaporate liquid in pan. Serves 6.

1 serving: 210 Calories; 1.3 g Total Fat (0.3 g Sat., trace Cholesterol); 218 mg Sodium; 4 g Protein; 47 g Carbohydrate; 7 g Dietary Fibre

CHOICES: 2 Grains & Starches; 3 Vegetables

Paré Pointer
The children of invisible parents wouldn't be much to look at.

Spicy Potato Bumps

Any combination of spices could be used for these, and they would still be as delicious!

Unpeeled medium baking potatoes	6	6
Olive oil	1 tbsp.	15 mL
Parsley flakes	2 tsp.	10 mL
Salt	1 1/2 tsp.	7 mL
Chili powder	1 tsp.	5 mL
Paprika	1 tsp.	5 mL
Dried thyme, crushed	1/2 tsp.	2 mL
Garlic powder	1/4 tsp.	1 mL
Cayenne pepper	1/8 tsp.	0.5 mL
Ground rosemary	1/16 tsp.	0.5 mL

Cut each potato in quarters lengthwise. Cut each quarter crosswise into 3 pieces. Toss potato with olive oil in large bowl.

Combine remaining 8 ingredients in small cup. Sprinkle over potato. Toss to coat. Spread on large greased baking sheet with sides. Bake, uncovered, in center of 425°F (220°C) oven. Cook for about 45 minutes, stirring twice, until browned and tender. Serves 6.

1 serving: 134 Calories; 2.6 g Total Fat (0.4 g Sat., 0 mg Cholesterol); 694 mg Sodium; 3 g Protein; 25 g Carbohydrate; 3 g Dietary Fibre

CHOICES: 1 1/2 Grains & Starches; 1/2 Fats

Pictured on page 126.

Crumbed Broccoli

Serve this spicy salad immediately after adding the crumbs.

Olive oil	2 tsp.	10 mL
Finely chopped jalapeño pepper, ribs and seeds removed (see Tip, page 105)	1 tbsp.	15 mL
Dry whole wheat bread crumbs (see Tip, page 80)	1/3 cup	75 mL
Garlic cloves, minced	3	3
Olive oil	2 tsp.	10 mL
Water	1/4 cup	60 mL
Head of broccoli, stems thinly sliced and florets cut bite size	1 1/2 lbs.	680 g

(continued on next page)

Side Dishes

Heat first amount of olive oil in small non-stick frying pan on medium. Sauté jalapeño for 30 seconds to 1 minute until slightly soft. Add bread crumbs. Sauté until crumbs are toasted and golden brown. Set aside.

Sauté garlic in second amount of olive oil until sizzling but not brown. Add water. Bring to a boil. Add broccoli stems on bottom of frying pan and florets on top. Cover. Heat on low for 5 to 6 minutes until broccoli is bright green and tender-crisp. Drain. Toss broccoli with crumb mixture in medium bowl. Makes 3 1/2 cups (875 mL).

2/3 cup (150 mL): 86 Calories; 3.7 g Total Fat (0.5 g Sat., 0.1 mg Cholesterol); 78 mg Sodium; 4 g Protein; 11 g Carbohydrate; 3 g Dietary Fibre

CHOICES: 1 Vegetables; 1/2 Fats

Cheese Spirals

Uses a container of Tomato Vegetable Sauce, page 118.

Lasagna noodles	8	8
Boiling water	3 qts.	3 L
Salt	1 tbsp.	15 mL
Grated part-skim mozzarella cheese	1/2 cup	125 mL
Light ricotta cheese	1/2 cup	125 mL
Grated light Parmesan cheese	2 tbsp.	30 mL
Dried marjoram, crushed	1/2 tsp.	2 mL
Dried sweet basil	1 tsp.	5 mL
Egg white (large), fork-beaten	1	1
Container of Tomato Vegetable Sauce (3 cups, 750 mL), page 118, thawed	1	1

Cook noodles in boiling water and salt in large uncovered pot or Dutch oven for 12 to 14 minutes until tender but firm. Drain. Rinse in cold water. Drain.

Combine next 3 ingredients in small bowl. Add next 3 ingredients. Mix. Spread cheese mixture along lengths of 8 cooked noodles. Roll up each, jelly roll style. Place seam side down in shallow baking dish.

Pour Tomato Vegetable Sauce over rolls. Cover. Bake in 350°F (175°C) oven for 30 to 40 minutes until bubbling and hot. Makes 8 rolls. Serves 4.

1 serving: 315 Calories; 7.7 g Total Fat (3.8 g Sat., 20.1 mg Cholesterol); 440 mg Sodium; 17 g Protein; 46 g Carbohydrate; 4 g Dietary Fibre

CHOICES: 2 Grains & Starches; 2 Vegetables; 1 Meat & Alternatives; 1/2 Fats

Pictured on page 126.

Creamy Garlic Spaghetti

A great side dish with just about any meat.

Box of whole wheat spaghetti	13 oz.	375 g
Boiling water	4 qts.	4 L
Salt	4 tsp.	20 mL
Chopped onion	1 1/2 cups	375 mL
Garlic cloves, minced	6	6
Olive oil	1 tbsp.	15 mL
All-purpose flour	1 tbsp.	15 mL
Vegetable (or chicken) bouillon powder	1 tsp.	5 mL
Water	3/4 cup	175 mL
Skim evaporated milk	1/4 cup	60 mL
Grated light Parmesan cheese	1/4 cup	60 mL
Chopped fresh parsley, for garnish		

Cook pasta in boiling water and salt in large uncovered pot or Dutch oven for 8 to 10 minutes until tender but firm. Drain well.

Sauté onion and garlic in olive oil in large non-stick frying pan for about 5 minutes until onion is golden and very soft. Sprinkle with flour and bouillon powder. Mix well. Gradually stir in water and milk. Heat and stir until bubbling. Cover. Simmer for about 30 minutes until thickened. Purée in blender. Makes 1 1/4 cups (300 mL).

Turn pasta into large bowl. Add garlic mixture and Parmesan cheese. Toss. Garnish with parsley. Makes 6 cups (1.5 L).

1 cup (250 mL): 287 Calories; 4 g Total Fat (0.9 g Sat., 2.2 mg Cholesterol); 206 mg Sodium; 13 g Protein; 54 g Carbohydrate; 8 g Dietary Fibre

CHOICES: 3 Grains & Starches; 1/2 Vegetables; 1/2 Fats

Paré Pointer

No wonder she dresses funny. She buys all her clothing when she's down in the dumps.

Caramelized Onion Strata

Good onion taste complements the tomatoes and crispy rye top.

Thinly sliced onion	2 cups	500 mL
Canola oil	1 tsp.	5 mL
Brown sugar, packed	1 tsp.	5 mL
Apple cider vinegar	1 tbsp.	15 mL
Rye bread cubes	6 cups	1.5 L
Medium Roma (plum) tomatoes, seeded and diced	4	4
Salt	1/2 tsp.	2 mL
Freshly ground pepper, sprinkle		
Dried whole oregano	1/2 tsp.	2 mL
No-salt herb seasoning	1 tsp.	5 mL
Grated light Swiss cheese	3/4 cup	175 mL
Frozen egg product, thawed (see Note)	1 cup	250 mL
Skim evaporated milk	3/4 cup	175 mL
Skim milk	3/4 cup	175 mL
Dry mustard	1/2 tsp.	2 mL
Grated light Swiss cheese	3/4 cup	175 mL

Sauté onion in canola oil on medium in large non-stick frying pan for about 5 minutes until softened. Stir in brown sugar and vinegar. Sauté for 4 to 5 minutes until deep golden.

Arrange 1/2 of bread cubes in greased 3 quart (3 L) shallow casserole. Layer with onion mixture and next 5 ingredients, in order. Sprinkle with first amount of cheese. Top with remaining bread cubes.

Beat next 4 ingredients in medium bowl. Pour evenly over bread cubes. Cover. Chill for several hours or overnight.

Bake, uncovered, in 325°F (160°C) oven for 1 hour. Sprinkle with second amount of cheese. Bake for about 15 minutes until set in center. Serves 6.

1 serving: 268 Calories; 6.5 g Total Fat (0.2 g Sat., 1.8 mg Cholesterol); 613 mg Sodium; 22 g Protein; 33 g Carbohydrate; 3 g Dietary Fibre

CHOICES: 1 Grains & Starches; 1 1/2 Vegetables; 1/2 Milk & Alternatives; 2 Meat & Alternatives

Note: 4 tbsp. (50 mL) = 1 large egg

Stuffed Tomatoes

Fresh flavour with a hint of tangy feta.

Large tomatoes	6	6
Chopped onion	1 cup	250 mL
Garlic cloves, minced	2	2
Olive oil	2 tsp.	10 mL
Chopped fresh mushrooms	1 cup	250 mL
Diced zucchini, with peel	1 1/2 cups	375 mL
Salt	1/2 tsp.	2 mL
Chopped fresh sweet basil (or 1 tsp., 5 mL, dried)	1 tbsp.	15 mL
Chopped fresh oregano leaves (or 1 tsp., 5 mL, dried)	1 tbsp.	15 mL
Whole wheat cracker crumbs	1/3 cup	75 mL
Crumbled feta cheese (about 4 oz., 113 g)	2/3 cup	150 g
Margarine	2 tsp.	10 mL
Whole wheat cracker crumbs	1/4 cup	60 mL
Finely chopped fresh parsley (or 1 tsp., 5 mL, flakes)	1 tbsp.	15 mL

Cut 1/4 inch (6 mm) slice from stem end of tomatoes. Scoop out pulp. Chop pulp finely. Set aside. Turn hollowed tomatoes upside down on paper towels to drain.

Sauté onion and garlic in olive oil in large non-stick frying pan on medium-high until onion is soft. Stir in mushrooms and zucchini. Sauté until soft.

Stir in next 4 ingredients. Add cheese. Add reserved tomato pulp. Stir. Makes 5 1/4 cups (1.3 L) filling. Fill tomato cavities.

Melt margarine in small saucepan. Stir in second amount of cracker crumbs and parsley. Sprinkle about 2 1/2 tsp. (12 mL) over each tomato. Place tomatoes in 9 x 13 inch (22 x 33 cm) baking pan. Pour in about 1/2 inch (12 mm) water. Bake, uncovered, in 350°F (175°C) oven for about 30 minutes until heated through. Makes 6 stuffed tomatoes.

1 stuffed tomato: 187 Calories; 10.3 g Total Fat (4.8 g Sat., 23.0 mg Cholesterol); 594 mg Sodium; 7 g Protein; 20 g Carbohydrate; 4 g Dietary Fibre

CHOICES: 2 Vegetables; 1/2 Meat & Alternatives; 2 Fats

Pictured on page 72.

Side Dishes

Creamy Mushroom Risotto

Contains threads of spinach throughout. The continuous stirring is what makes it creamy.

Olive oil	2 tsp.	10 mL
Sliced fresh mushrooms	3 cups	750 mL
Garlic clove, minced	1	1
Dried sweet basil	1 1/2 tsp.	7 mL
Freshly ground pepper, sprinkle		
Water	1 1/2 cups	375 mL
Vegetable bouillon powder	1 tbsp.	15 mL
Short grain white (or arborio) rice	1 1/2 cups	375 mL
Water	1 1/4 cups	300 mL
White (or alcohol-free) wine	1/4 cup	60 mL
Skim milk	1/4 cup	60 mL
Fresh spinach leaves, lightly packed, cut chiffonade (see Tip, below)	3 cups	750 mL
Chopped toasted pine nuts (see Tip, page 111)	1/3 cup	75 mL
Freshly grated Parmesan cheese	1/4 cup	60 mL

Heat olive oil in large non-stick frying pan. Add next 4 ingredients. Heat and stir on medium-high for about 10 minutes until liquid is evaporated and mushrooms are browned.

Add next 3 ingredients. Bring to a boil. Heat and stir until almost all of water is absorbed.

Add second amount of water, 1/4 cup (60 mL) at a time, while stirring. Allow water to absorb with each addition.

Add wine. Heat and stir until absorbed. Stir in milk and spinach. Heat and stir until milk is absorbed and spinach is soft. Turn into warm serving bowl. Sprinkle with nuts and cheese. Makes 5 cups (1.25 L). Serves 6.

1 serving: 304 Calories; 8.4 g Total Fat (2.0 g Sat., 3.9 mg Cholesterol); 412 mg Sodium; 10 g Protein; 47 g Carbohydrate; 3 g Dietary Fibre

CHOICES: 3 Grains & Starches; 1 Fats

 tip To cut chiffonade: stack leaves, roll tightly lengthwise and then thinly slice crosswise.

Roasted Veggies

Love that sweet roasted flavour. Make use of the many different salt-free herb preparations to change the flavour to suit your tastes.

Red baby potatoes (about 10), halved	1 lb.	454 g
Baby carrots (about 8 oz., 225 g)	1 3/4 cups	425 mL
Large cauliflower florets (about 10 oz., 285 g)	2 1/4 cups	550 mL
Parsnips, cut into 1 inch (2.5 cm) thick slices (about 8 oz., 225 g)	4	4
Olive oil	1 tbsp.	15 mL
Water	1 tbsp.	15 mL
Garlic clove, minced (optional)	1	1
No-salt Italian herb seasoning	1 tbsp.	15 mL
Salt	1/2 tsp.	2 mL
Freshly ground pepper, sprinkle		

Combine first 4 ingredients in lightly greased 9 x 13 inch (22 x 33 cm) pan.

Combine remaining 6 ingredients in small dish. Pour over vegetable mixture. Toss well. Bake, covered, in 450°F (230°C) oven for 30 minutes. Stir. Bake, uncovered, for 30 minutes until vegetables are tender and starting to turn brown. Serves 4.

1 serving: 210 Calories; 4 g Total Fat (0.6 g Sat., 0 mg Cholesterol); 384 mg Sodium; 5 g Protein; 41 g Carbohydrate; 7 g Dietary Fibre

CHOICES: 1 1/2 Grains & Starches; 4 Vegetables; 1/2 Fats

Paré Pointer

Fish hate tennis because they don't want to be around the net.

Side Dishes

Tomatoes Provençale

Make this dish when tomatoes are fresh out of your garden.

Whole wheat bread slices, torn up	2	2
Garlic clove, minced	1	1
Ground rosemary	1/8 tsp.	0.5 mL
Salt	1/8 tsp.	0.5 mL
Freshly ground pepper, generous sprinkle		
Medium tomatoes	4	4
Olive oil	2 tsp.	10 mL

Process first 5 ingredients in blender or food processor until crumbled.

Cut tomatoes into thick slices. Place in rows, slightly overlapping, in 9 × 13 inch (22 × 33 cm) pan or shallow 2 quart (2 L) baking dish. Brush surface with olive oil. Sprinkle with crumb mixture. Bake, uncovered, in 400°F (205°C) oven for 10 minutes until crumbs are browned and slightly crisp. Serves 6.

1 serving: 54 Calories; 2 g Total Fat (0.3 g Sat., 0.3 mg Cholesterol); 116 mg Sodium; 2 g Protein; 9 g Carbohydrate; 2 g Dietary Fibre

CHOICES: 1/2 Grains & Starches

Mashed Garlic Potatoes

Boost the flavour of ordinary mashed potatoes in one easy step!

Potatoes, peeled and cut into large chunks	1 1/2 lbs.	680 g
Garlic cloves, cut in half	6	6
Salt	1 tsp.	5 mL
Boiling water		
Skim evaporated milk	1/3 cup	75 mL
Freshly ground pepper, sprinkle		

Cook potatoes with garlic and salt in boiling water in medium saucepan for 12 minutes until tender. Drain, reserving 1/4 cup (60 mL) potato water.

Mash potato, reserved potato water, evaporated milk and pepper until smooth and fluffy. Makes 3 1/2 cups (875 mL). Serves 6.

1 serving: 106 Calories; 0.2 g Total Fat (0.1 g Sat., 0.5 mg Cholesterol); 25 mg Sodium; 4 g Protein; 23 g Carbohydrate; 2 g Dietary Fibre

CHOICES: 1 1/2 Grains & Starches

Side Dishes

Rice Pilaf

Nice toasted grain flavour. Try the variation for even more fibre.

Chopped onion	1/2 cup	125 mL
Sliced fresh mushrooms	1 cup	250 mL
Canola oil	2 tsp.	10 mL
Long grain white rice	1/2 cup	125 mL
Bulgur wheat	1/2 cup	125 mL
Can of condensed chicken broth	10 oz.	284 mL
Water	3/4 cup	175 mL
Chopped fresh parsley (optional)	1 tbsp.	15 mL

Sauté onion and mushrooms in canola oil in large frying pan until soft. Add rice and bulgur. Sauté for about 10 minutes until rice is toasted. Turn into medium saucepan.

Stir in broth and water. Bring to a boil. Reduce heat. Cover. Simmer for 20 minutes until liquid is absorbed.

Stir in parsley. Makes 3 cups (750 mL).

1/2 cup (125 mL): 139 Calories; 2.4 g Total Fat (0.3 g Sat., 0.5 mg Cholesterol); 318 mg Sodium; 5 g Protein; 25 g Carbohydrate; 3 g Dietary Fibre

CHOICES: 1 1/2 Grains & Starches; 1/2 Fats

Variation: For more colour and fibre, stir in 1 cup (250 mL) hot cooked peas just before serving.

Barley Side Dish

Wonderful barley flavour and chewy texture.

Chopped onion	1/2 cup	125 mL
Chopped celery	1/2 cup	125 mL
Canola oil	2 tsp.	10 mL
Pearl barley	1 cup	250 mL
Boiling water	3 1/2 cups	875 mL
Beef bouillon powder	1 tbsp.	15 mL
Medium carrot, grated	1	1
Chopped green onion (or chives)	2 tbsp.	30 mL

(continued on next page)

138 Side Dishes

Sauté onion and celery in canola oil in large frying pan until soft. Add barley. Sauté for about 10 minutes until barley is toasted. Turn into medium saucepan.

Stir in next 3 ingredients. Bring to a boil. Reduce heat. Cover. Simmer for 30 to 35 minutes until liquid is absorbed. Stir in green onion. Makes 4 cups (1 L).

3/4 cup (175 mL): 146 Calories; 2.5 g Total Fat (0.4 g Sat., 0.2 mg Cholesterol); 316 mg Sodium; 5 g Protein; 27 g Carbohydrate; 6 g Dietary Fibre

CHOICES: 1 1/2 Grains & Starches; 1/2 Vegetables; 1/2 Meat & Alternatives; 1/2 Fats

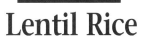

Lentil Rice

Exotic Middle Eastern influences in this tasty dish.
Makes a big batch and rewarms wonderfully for lunches at work.

Water	12 cups	3 L
Green lentils	2 cups	500 mL
Bay leaves	5	5
Dried crushed chilies	1/4 tsp.	1 mL
Salt	1 tsp.	5 mL
Freshly ground pepper	1 tsp.	5 mL
Long grain white rice	1 cup	250 mL
Pickled hot peppers, chopped (optional)	1/2 cup	125 mL

Combine first 6 ingredients in large pot or Dutch oven. Cover. Simmer for 40 minutes until lentils are tender but firm.

Stir in rice. Bring to a boil. Cover. Simmer for 15 to 20 minutes until rice is tender. Drain any remaining liquid. Stir in hot pepper. Makes 8 cups (2 L).

1/2 cup (125 mL): 131 Calories; 0.3 g Total Fat (0.1 g Sat., 0 mg Cholesterol); 173 mg Sodium; 8 g Protein; 24 g Carbohydrate; 3 g Dietary Fibre

CHOICES: 1 Grains & Starches; 1 Meat & Alternatives

Pictured on page 72.

Investing in good non-stick cookware makes it easier to use less oil to keep food from sticking when cooking. Oive and canola oils add taste and are low in saturated fats.

Italian Potato Casserole

Moist and tender with herb and pepper aftertaste.

Medium onion, sliced	1	1
Garlic clove, minced	1	1
Olive oil	1 tsp.	5 mL
Skim evaporated milk	1 cup	250 mL
All-purpose flour	3 tbsp.	50 mL
Prepared mustard	2 tsp.	10 mL
Salt	1/2 tsp.	2 mL
Dried sweet basil	1/2 tsp.	2 mL
Granulated sugar	1/4 tsp.	1 mL
Dried whole oregano	1/8 tsp.	0.5 mL
Unpeeled medium new potatoes, thinly sliced (about 4 cups, 1 L)	4	4
Freshly ground pepper	1/8 tsp.	0.5 mL
Medium Roma (plum) tomatoes, sliced 1/4 inch (6 mm) thick	4	4
Grated light Parmesan cheese	1 tbsp.	15 mL

Sauté onion and garlic in olive oil in medium non-stick frying pan until onion is soft.

Combine evaporated milk and flour in small bowl until smooth. Slowly add to onion, stirring constantly, until boiling and thickened. Stir in next 5 ingredients.

Arrange 1/2 of potato in greased 2 quart (2 L) casserole. Sprinkle with pepper. Layer with 1/2 of tomato. Cover with 1/2 of onion mixture. Repeat layers. Sprinkle with Parmesan cheese. Cover. Bake in 375°F (190°C) oven for 45 minutes. Remove cover. Bake for 20 to 30 minutes until golden brown and potato is soft. Makes 5 cups (1.25 L).

3/4 cup (175 mL): 161 Calories; 1.6 g Total Fat (0.3 g Sat., 2.0 mg Cholesterol); 337 mg Sodium; 8 g Protein; 31 g Carbohydrate; 3 g Dietary Fibre

CHOICES: 1 Grains & Starches; 1 Vegetables; 1/2 Milk & Alternatives

Pictured on page 143.

Barley And Rice Pilaf

The barley makes it slightly chewy. Good blend of flavours,
but you can add up to a teaspoon (5 mL) of your favourite
no-salt herb seasoning for more of a flavour burst.

Pearl barley	3/4 cup	175 mL
Long grain brown rice	3/4 cup	175 mL
Canola oil	1 tbsp.	15 mL
Chopped onion	1 cup	250 mL
Chopped celery, with leaves	1 cup	250 mL
Water	3 1/2 cups	875 mL
Vegetable bouillon powder	1 tbsp.	15 mL
Coarsely grated carrot	1/2 cup	125 mL
Diced green pepper	1/2 cup	125 mL
Diced red pepper	1/2 cup	125 mL
Diced yellow or orange pepper	1/2 cup	125 mL
Garlic powder	1/4 tsp.	1 mL
Chopped fresh parsley (or 2 tsp., 10 mL, flakes)	3 tbsp.	50 mL
Salt	1 1/2 tsp.	7 mL
Pepper	1/2 tsp.	2 mL

Sauté barley and rice in canola oil in large heavy-bottomed saucepan for about 8 minutes until starting to turn golden brown.

Add onion and celery. Sauté for 3 to 4 minutes until celery is tender-crisp. Add next 3 ingredients. Bring to a boil. Reduce heat. Cover. Simmer for 40 minutes.

Stir in remaining 7 ingredients. Cover. Simmer for 20 to 30 minutes until water is absorbed and barley is tender. Makes 6 cups (1.5 L).

1/2 cup (125 mL): 115 Calories; 2 g Total Fat (0.3 g Sat., 0.1 mg Cholesterol); 502 mg Sodium; 3 g Protein; 22 g Carbohydrate; 3 g Dietary Fibre

CHOICES: 1 Grains & Starches; 1/2 Vegetables

Pictured on page 143.

Cold Dressed Asparagus

This is a great make-ahead recipe. It suits an elegant
dinner party, an outdoor barbecue or a potluck.

Medium tomato, quartered	1	1
Green onion, cut into 1 inch (2.5 cm) pieces	1	1
Garlic cloves	2	2
Red wine vinegar	3 tbsp.	50 mL
Liquid honey	1 tbsp.	15 mL
Chopped fresh parsley	1 tbsp.	15 mL
Olive oil	1 tbsp.	15 mL
Anchovy paste	2 tsp.	10 mL
Paprika	1 tsp.	5 mL
Salt	1/2 tsp.	2 mL
Fresh asparagus, trimmed of tough ends	1 lb.	454 g
Very thinly sliced red onion	1 1/2 cups	375 mL
Chopped pitted ripe olives (optional)	2 tbsp.	30 mL

Process first 10 ingredients in blender for about 1 minute until smooth. Chill for 1 hour to blend flavours. Makes 1 1/4 cups (300 mL) dressing.

Steam asparagus for 4 to 5 minutes until tender-crisp. Drain. Rinse in cold water until completely cool. Drain well.

Arrange asparagus and onion on small platter. Scatter with olives. Drizzle dressing over top. Serve chilled or at room temperature. Serves 8.

1 serving: 59 Calories; 2.2 g Total Fat (0.3 g Sat., 1.5 mg Cholesterol); 238 mg Sodium; 3 g Protein; 9 g Carbohydrate; 2 g Dietary Fibre

CHOICES: 1 Vegetables, 1/2 Meat & Alternatives

Pictured at right.

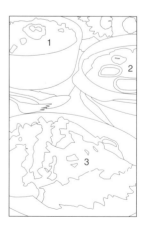

1. Barley And Rice Pilaf, page 141
2. Italian Potato Casserole, page 140
3. Cold Dressed Asparagus, above

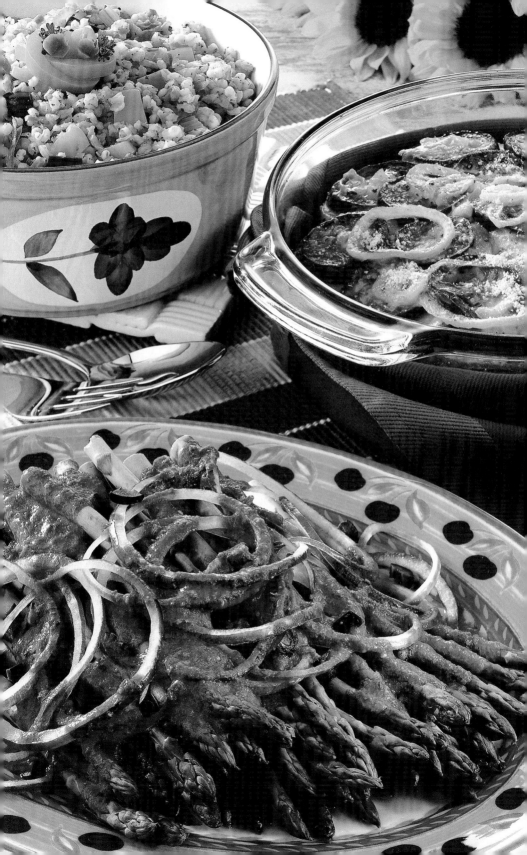

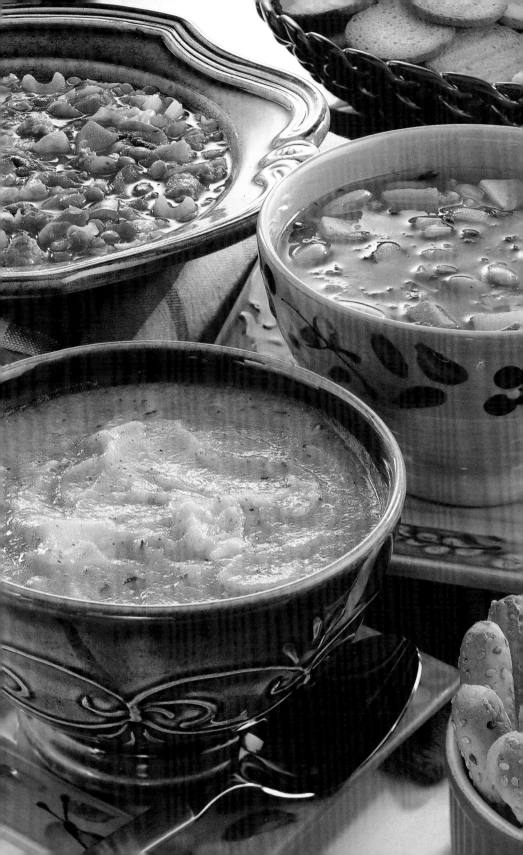

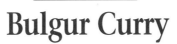

Bulgur Curry

Such a warm, pretty colour—and it tastes good too. Makes an impressive buffet dish.

Large onion, chopped	1	1
Chopped fresh mushrooms	1 cup	250 mL
Diced red or green pepper	1 cup	250 mL
Olive oil	2 tsp.	10 mL
Curry paste (available in Asian section of grocery store)	1 tsp.	5 mL
Dark raisins	1/3 cup	75 mL
Water	3 cups	750 mL
Chicken bouillon powder	1 tbsp.	15 mL
Bulgur wheat	1 1/4 cups	300 mL
Chopped fresh parsley (or 1 tbsp., 15 mL, flakes)	1/4 cup	60 mL

Sauté first 3 ingredients in olive oil in large saucepan on medium for about 10 minutes until onion is soft and liquid is evaporated.

Stir in curry paste and raisins. Add next 3 ingredients. Bring to a boil. Reduce heat. Cover. Simmer for about 20 minutes until liquid is absorbed.

Stir in parsley before serving. Makes 5 cups (1.25 L).

1/2 cup (125 mL): 99 Calories; 1.5 g Total Fat (0.2 g Sat., 0.1 mg Cholesterol); 200 mg Sodium; 3 g Protein; 20 g Carbohydrate; 4 g Dietary Fibre

CHOICES: 1 Grains & Starches; 1/2 Vegetables

Pictured on page 126.

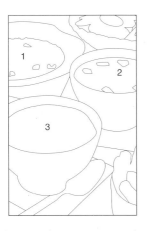

1. Lentil Soup, page 148
2. White Bean Soup, page 146
3. Curried Zucchini Chowder, page 147

White Bean Soup

The list of ingredients might seem lengthy, but you can
be eating hot soup in an hour from start to finish.

Sliced leeks (halved lengthwise and rinsed well)	1 cup	250 mL
Chopped celery heart and leaves	1 cup	250 mL
Garlic cloves, minced	2	2
Olive oil	2 tsp.	10 mL
Diced carrot	1 cup	250 mL
Diced potato	1 cup	250 mL
Can of Italian-spiced diced tomatoes, with juice, puréed	14 oz.	398 mL
Water	4 cups	1 L
Chicken bouillon powder	1 tbsp.	15 mL
Hot pepper sauce	1/2 tsp.	2 mL
Celery seed	1/2 tsp.	2 mL
Salt	1/2 tsp.	2 mL
Freshly ground pepper	1/8 tsp.	0.5 mL
Dried sweet basil (optional)	1/2 tsp.	2 mL
Fennel seed, crushed (optional)	1/4 tsp.	1 mL
Can of white kidney beans, drained and rinsed	19 oz.	540 mL
Shredded fresh spinach leaves, packed	1 cup	250 mL
Finely chopped fresh parsley (or 1 tsp., 5 mL, flakes)	1 tbsp.	15 mL

Sauté first 3 ingredients in olive oil in large uncovered pot or Dutch oven until softened.

Add next 9 ingredients. Bring to a boil. Reduce heat. Simmer, partially covered, for 10 to 15 minutes until carrot and potato are tender.

Stir in remaining 5 ingredients. Cover. Simmer for 5 minutes until spinach is softened. Makes 8 cups (2 L).

1 cup (250 mL): 104 Calories; 1.7 g Total Fat (0.3 g Sat., 0.2 mg Cholesterol); 655 mg Sodium; 5 g Protein; 19 g Carbohydrate; 2 g Dietary Fibre

CHOICES: 1 1/2 Vegetables

Pictured on page 144.

Curried Zucchini Chowder

The curry flavour is mild but a swirl of yogurt, sour cream or cream in the soup at serving time will mellow the flavour even more.

Chopped onion	1 cup	250 mL
Garlic clove, minced	1	1
Margarine	2 tsp.	10 mL
Curry paste (available in Asian section of grocery store)	1/2 tsp.	2 mL
Grated zucchini (about 3 medium), with peel	4 cups	1 L
Diced potato	3 cups	750 mL
Water	3 1/4 cups	800 mL
Vegetable bouillon powder	2 tbsp.	30 mL
Bay leaf	1	1
Freshly ground pepper	1/4 tsp.	1 mL
Ground cumin	1/16 tsp.	0.5 mL

Sauté onion and garlic in margarine in large uncovered pot or Dutch oven until onion is very soft and turning golden brown. Stir in curry paste. Sauté for 1 minute.

Stir in remaining 7 ingredients. Heat on medium, partially covered, for 1 hour. Remove and discard bay leaf. Remove and reserve 2 cups (500 mL) vegetable mixture. Process remaining vegetable mixture with hand blender or in batches in blender until smooth. Combine reserved and puréed vegetable mixture in same pot. Makes 7 cups (1.75 L).

1 cup (250 mL): 92 Calories; 1.6 g Total Fat (0.4 g Sat., 0.3 mg Cholesterol); 530 mg Sodium; 3 g Protein; 18 g Carbohydrate; 3 g Dietary Fibre

CHOICES: 1 Grains & Starches; 1 Vegetables

Pictured on page 144.

Paré Pointer

In the afternoons, kings and queens drink royal-tea.

Lentil Soup

This thick, hearty soup is a meal in itself. Serve with crusty bread or buns.

Lean ground chicken	8 oz.	225 g
Chopped onion	1/2 cup	125 mL
Sliced fresh mushrooms	1 cup	250 mL
Canola oil	2 tsp.	10 mL
Water	5 cups	1.25 L
Can of diced tomatoes, with juice	28 oz.	796 mL
Chopped cabbage	2 cups	500 mL
Sliced celery	1 cup	250 mL
Diced carrot	1 cup	250 mL
Diced green (or other) pepper	1/2 cup	125 mL
Bay leaves	2	2
Vegetable bouillon powder	2 tsp.	10 mL
Worcestershire sauce	1/2 tsp.	2 mL
Dried thyme leaves	1/2 tsp.	2 mL
Green lentils	3/4 cup	175 mL

Sauté first 3 ingredients in canola oil in large uncovered pot or Dutch oven until starting to brown. Drain.

Add remaining 11 ingredients to ground chicken mixture. Bring to a boil. Reduce heat. Partially cover. Simmer for 45 minutes until lentils and vegetables are tender. Makes 10 cups (2.5 L).

1 cup (250 mL): 120 Calories; 1.7 g Total Fat (0.2 g Sat., 13.1 mg Cholesterol); 288 mg Sodium; 11 g Protein; 16 g Carbohydrate; 4 g Dietary Fibre

CHOICES: 1 1/2 Vegetables; 1 Meat & Alternatives

Pictured on page 144.

Paré Pointer

Saturday and Sunday are very strong days.
The other five are weekdays.

Chilled Vegetable Soup

A refreshing soup that uses up those bits of fresh herbs and vegetables in the refrigerator!

Vegetable cocktail juice	2 1/2 cups	625 mL
Diced fresh tomato	2 cups	500 mL
Water	1 cup	250 mL
Diced red or green pepper	1 cup	250 mL
Diced cucumber, with peel	1 cup	250 mL
Chopped green onion	1/2 cup	125 mL
Chopped fresh chives (or 1 tsp., 5 mL, dried)	1 tbsp.	15 mL
Chopped fresh oregano leaves (or 1/2 tsp., 2 mL, dried)	1 tbsp.	15 mL
Chopped fresh sweet basil (or 2 tsp., 10 mL, dried)	2 tbsp.	30 mL
Lemon juice	2 tbsp.	30 mL

Light sour cream, for garnish
Hot pepper sauce, for garnish

Combine first 10 ingredients in large bowl. Chill for several hours or overnight.

Purée 1/2 in blender or food processor. Return to bowl. Stir. Spoon into individual serving bowls. Add dollop of sour cream and dash of pepper sauce if desired. Makes 7 3/4 cups (1.9 L).

1 cup (250 mL): 34 Calories; 0.3 g Total Fat (trace Sat., 0 mg Cholesterol); 306 mg Sodium; 1 g Protein; 8 g Carbohydrate; 1 g Dietary Fibre

CHOICES: 1 1/2 Vegetables

 tip   Generally, when substituting dried for fresh herbs, use about 1/4 of the amount requested. For example, you would use 3/4 tsp. (4 mL) dried where the recipe called for 1 tsp (15 mL) of fresh herbs.

Turtle Bean Soup

Gentle heat from the chili powder and the hot pepper sauce.

Chopped onion	1 cup	250 mL
Canola oil	2 tsp.	10 mL
Garlic cloves, minced	2	2
Medium red pepper, diced	1	1
Water	4 cups	1 L
Vegetable bouillon powder	2 tbsp.	30 mL
Can of black beans, drained and rinsed	19 oz.	540 mL
Chili powder	1 1/2 tsp.	7 mL
Bay leaf	1	1
Dried whole marjoram (or oregano), crushed	1/2 tsp.	2 mL
Dried sweet basil	1 tsp.	5 mL
Kernel corn, fresh or frozen	1/2 cup	125 mL
Lime juice	2 tsp.	10 mL
Hot pepper sauce	1/2 tsp.	2 mL
Cooked mashed potato	1 cup	250 mL
Chopped fresh parsley	1/4 cup	60 mL
Chopped fresh cilantro (optional)	1 tbsp.	15 mL
Non-fat plain yogurt (or light sour cream), optional		
Sliced green onion (optional)		

Sauté onion in canola oil in large uncovered pot or Dutch oven until soft. Add garlic and red pepper. Sauté for about 2 minutes until pepper is soft.

Stir in next 11 ingredients. Cover. Simmer on medium-low for 40 minutes.

Remove and discard bay leaf. Stir in parsley and cilantro (see Note). Spoon into individual serving bowls. Top with a dollop of yogurt and sprinkle of green onion. Makes 6 cups (1.5 L).

1 cup (250 mL): 148 Calories; 2.5 g Total Fat (0.4 g Sat., 0.4 mg Cholesterol); 711 mg Sodium; 6 g Protein; 27 g Carbohydrate; 4 g Dietary Fibre

CHOICES: 1 Grains & Starches; 1 1/2 Vegetables; 1/2 Meat & Alternatives

Note: To make a thicker soup, purée 3 cups (750 mL) soup in blender. Return to pot. Heat through.

Barley Vegetable Soup

Thick, hearty soup warms the insides on a cold winter day.

Water	2 qts.	2 L
Pearl barley	1 cup	250 mL
Chopped onion	1 cup	250 mL
Chopped celery	1 cup	250 mL
Diced carrot	1 cup	250 mL
Vegetable bouillon powder	2 tbsp.	30 mL
Medium potatoes, peeled and diced	2	2
Worcestershire sauce	1 1/2 tsp.	7 mL
Dried sweet basil	1 1/2 tsp.	7 mL
Parsley flakes	1 tsp.	5 mL
Freshly ground pepper, sprinkle		
Vegetable cocktail juice	1 cup	250 mL
All-purpose flour	2 tbsp.	30 mL

Put first 6 ingredients into large uncovered pot or Dutch oven. Cover. Simmer for 30 minutes.

Add next 5 ingredients. Cover. Simmer for 15 minutes until potato is tender.

Whisk vegetable juice into flour in small bowl until smooth. Stir into soup. Simmer for 1 minute until slightly thickened. Makes 10 1/2 cups (2.6 L).

1 cup (250 mL): 117 Calories; 0.6 g Total Fat (0.2 g Sat., 0.2 mg Cholesterol); 456 mg Sodium; 4 g Protein; 26 g Carbohydrate; 4 g Dietary Fibre

CHOICES: 1 Grains & Starches; 1 Vegetables

 If your homemade soup is too salty, drop a peeled potato into the pot and remove just before serving.

Roasted Garlic Soup

*Roast some garlic the next time you have your oven on to make
this special soup. Serve small amounts for an elegant first course.*

Large heads of garlic (not individual cloves)	4	4
Olive oil	2 tsp.	10 mL
Water	1/4 cup	60 mL
Chopped onion	2/3 cup	150 mL
Olive oil	2 tsp.	10 mL
Peeled and diced potato	3 cups	750 mL
Can of condensed chicken broth	10 oz.	284 mL
Water	2/3 cup	150 mL
Dried tarragon	1 tsp.	5 mL
Granulated sugar	1 tsp.	5 mL
Salt	1/2 tsp.	2 mL
Cayenne pepper	1/8 tsp.	0.5 mL
Can of skim evaporated milk	13 1/2 oz.	385 mL
All-purpose flour	2 tbsp.	30 mL
White (or alcohol-free) wine	1/2 cup	125 mL

Remove loose papery skin from garlic heads, being careful not separate or peel
individual cloves. Cut tops off garlic heads to barely expose tops of some cloves.
Place in garlic baker or small pie plate. Drizzle 1/2 tsp. (2 mL) of first amount
of olive oil over each garlic head. Drizzle first amount of water into baking dish.
Cover tightly with lid or foil. Bake in 350°F (175°C) oven for about 45 minutes
until garlic cloves are soft and golden. Cool enough to handle. Squeeze out cloves
into small bowl.

Sauté onion in second amount of olive oil in large saucepan until soft. Add next
3 ingredients. Cover. Simmer for about 15 minutes until potato is very tender.

Stir in roasted garlic. Add next 4 ingredients. Purée in blender or food processor until
smooth. Return to saucepan. Bring to a boil.

Stir evaporated milk into flour in small bowl until smooth. Add to soup. Heat and
stir on medium until slightly thickened. Add wine. Stir. Makes 6 cups (1.5 L).

*1 cup (250 mL): 238 Calories; 4 g Total Fat (0.7 g Sat., 3.0 mg Cholesterol); 632 mg Sodium;
12 g Protein; 37 g Carbohydrate; 2 g Dietary Fibre*

CHOICES: 1 Grains & Starches; 2 Vegetables; 1/2 Milk & Alternatives; 1/2 Fats

Minestrone Soup

Thick and chunky with a rich-tasting broth. A hearty meal with some bread or buns.

Container of Tomato Vegetable Sauce (3 cups, 750 mL), page 118, thawed	1	1
Water	4 cups	1 L
Sliced celery	1/2 cup	125 mL
Finely diced carrot	1/2 cup	125 mL
Chopped cabbage	1 cup	250 mL
Beef bouillon powder	2 tsp.	10 mL
Granulated sugar	1 tsp.	5 mL
No-salt garlic and herb seasoning	1 tsp.	5 mL
Dried crushed chilies	1/8 tsp.	0.5 mL
Can of kidney beans, drained and rinsed	14 oz.	398 mL
Whole wheat elbow macaroni	1/2 cup	125 mL

Grated Parmesan cheese (optional)

Combine Tomato Vegetable Sauce and water in large saucepan. Bring to a boil. Add next 7 ingredients. Cover. Simmer for 30 minutes.

Stir in beans and pasta. Cover. Bring to a boil. Cook for 10 minutes, stirring twice, until pasta is tender.

Sprinkle individual servings with Parmesan cheese. Makes 7 cups (1.75 L).

1 cup (250 mL): 120 Calories; 1.3 g Total Fat (0.2 g Sat., 0.1 mg Cholesterol); 406 mg Sodium; 6 g Protein; 24 g Carbohydrate; 6 g Dietary Fibre

CHOICES: 1/2 Grains & Starches; 2 Vegetables

 tip To keep garlic bulbs from sprouting, softening and drying out, store in a container in the freezer. To easily peel a clove at a time, heat on high (100%) for 30 seconds in microwave.

Bean And Bacon Soup

Rich, warm flavour from bacon. Hearty comfort food.

Chopped onion	2/3 cup	150 mL
Chopped celery	2/3 cup	150 mL
Garlic cloves, minced	2	2
Canola oil	2 tsp.	10 mL
Canadian back bacon, diced	2 oz.	57 g
Water	5 cups	1.25 L
Vegetable bouillon powder	1 tbsp.	15 mL
Sliced carrot	1 cup	250 mL
Peeled, diced potato	2 cups	500 mL
Bay leaves	2	2
Can of mixed beans, drained and rinsed	19 oz.	540 mL
Can of baked beans in tomato sauce	14 oz.	398 mL

Sauté first 3 ingredients in canola oil in large uncovered pot or Dutch oven until very soft. Add bacon. Sauté until starting to brown.

Add next 5 ingredients. Bring to a boil. Cover. Simmer for 25 minutes until potato is very tender and breaking up.

Stir in both beans. Heat, uncovered, for about 10 minutes until soup is thickened. Remove and discard bay leaves. Makes 8 cups (2 L).

1 cup (250 mL): 160 Calories; 2.4 g Total Fat (0.4 g Sat., 3.7 mg Cholesterol); 626 mg Sodium; 8 g Protein; 29 g Carbohydrate; 8 g Dietary Fibre

CHOICES: 1 1/2 Grains & Starches; 1/2 Vegetables; 1 Meat & Alternatives

Measurement Tables

Throughout this book measurements are given in Conventional and Metric measure. To compensate for differences between the two measurements due to rounding, a full metric measure is not always used. The cup used is the standard 8 fluid ounce. Temperature is given in degrees Fahrenheit and Celsius. Baking pan measurements are in inches and centimetres as well as quarts and litres. An exact metric conversion is given below as well as the working equivalent (Metric Standard Measure).

Spoons

Conventional Measure	Metric Exact Conversion Millilitre (mL)	Metric Standard Measure Millilitre (mL)
1/8 teaspoon (tsp.)	0.6 mL	0.5 mL
1/4 teaspoon (tsp.)	1.2 mL	1 mL
1/2 teaspoon (tsp.)	2.4 mL	2 mL
1 teaspoon (tsp.)	4.7 mL	5 mL
2 teaspoons (tsp.)	9.4 mL	10 mL
1 tablespoon (tbsp.)	14.2 mL	15 mL

Cups

Conventional Measure	Metric Exact Conversion Millilitre (mL)	Metric Standard Measure Millilitre (mL)
1/4 cup (4 tbsp.)	56.8 mL	60 mL
1/3 cup (5 1/3 tbsp.)	75.6 mL	75 mL
1/2 cup (8 tbsp.)	113.7 mL	125 mL
2/3 cup (10 2/3 tbsp.)	151.2 mL	150 mL
3/4 cup (12 tbsp.)	170.5 mL	175 mL
1 cup (16 tbsp.)	227.3 mL	250 mL
4 1/2 cups	1022.9 mL	1000 mL (1 L)

Oven Temperatures

Fahrenheit (°F)	Celsius (°C)
175°	80°
200°	95°
225°	110°
250°	120°
275°	140°
300°	150°
325°	160°
350°	175°
375°	190°
400°	205°
425°	220°
450°	230°
475°	240°
500°	260°

Dry Measurements

Conventional Measure Ounces (oz.)	Metric Exact Conversion Grams (g)	Metric Standard Measure Grams (g)
1 oz.	28.3 g	28 g
2 oz.	56.7 g	57 g
3 oz.	85.0 g	85 g
4 oz.	113.4 g	125 g
5 oz.	141.7 g	140 g
6 oz.	170.1 g	170 g
7 oz.	198.4 g	200 g
8 oz.	226.8 g	250 g
16 oz.	453.6 g	500 g
32 oz.	907.2 g	1000 g (1 kg)

Pans

Conventional Inches	Metric Centimetres
8x8 inch	20x20 cm
9x9 inch	22x22 cm
9x13 inch	22x33 cm
10x15 inch	25x38 cm
11x17 inch	28x43 cm
8x2 inch round	20x5 cm
9x2 inch round	22x5 cm
10x4 1/2 inch tube	25x11 cm
8x4x3 inch loaf	20x10x7.5 cm
9x5x3 inch loaf	22x12.5x7.5 cm

Casseroles

CANADA & BRITAIN		UNITED STATES	
Standard Size Casserole	Exact Metric Measure	Standard Size Casserole	Exact Metric Measure
1 qt. (5 cups)	1.13 L	1 qt. (4 cups)	900 mL
1 1/2 qts. (7 1/2 cups)	1.69 L	1 1/2 qts. (6 cups)	1.35 L
2 qts. (10 cups)	2.25 L	2 qts. (8 cups)	1.8 L
2 1/2 qts. (12 1/2 cups)	2.81 L	2 1/2 qts. (10 cups)	2.25 L
3 qts. (15 cups)	3.38 L	3 qts. (12 cups)	2.7 L
4 qts. (20 cups)	4.5 L	4 qts. (16 cups)	3.6 L
5 qts. (25 cups)	5.63 L	5 qts. (20 cups)	4.5 L

Tip Index

Recipe Index